TODAY WAS A GOOD DAY

*A Collection of Essays
From The Heart Of A Neurosurgeon*

by

Edward Benzel

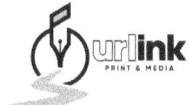

Today Was A Good Day

Copyright © 2024 by Edward Benzel. All rights reserved.

No part of this publication may be reproduced, stored in a retrieval system or transmitted in any way by any means, electronic, mechanical, photocopy, recording or otherwise without the prior permission of the author except as provided by USA copyright law.

The opinions expressed by the author are not necessarily those of URLink Print and Media.

1603 Capitol Ave., Suite 310 Cheyenne, Wyoming USA 82001
1-888-980-6523 | admin@urlinkpublishing.com

URLink Print and Media is committed to excellence in the publishing industry.

Book design copyright © 2024 by URLink Print and Media. All rights reserved.

Published in the United States of America
ISBN 978-1-68486-887-2 (Paperback)
ISBN 978-1-68486-895-7 (Digital)

31.07.24

CONTENTS

Foreword vii

Preface ix

SECTION ONE: INTRODUCTION
I THINK, THEREFORE, I AM:
CRAFTING A BETTER VERSION OF OURSELVES 1

    Essay 1:   Empathy, A Foundational Attribute

    Essay 2:   Respect

    Essay 3:   Stress and Stress Recovery

    Essay 4:   Leadership

    Essay 5:   Fatigue, or Is It Burnout?

    Essay 6:   Competence

    Essay 7:   The Humility Button

    Essay 8:   Optimism vs. Pessimism, The Choice Is Yours

    Essay 9:   Self and Social Awareness

    Essay 10: Celebrate

    Essay 11: Experience

    Essay 12: What the People of Ukraine Have Taught Us

SECTION TWO: INTRODUCTION
TODAY WAS A GOOD DAY 31

    Essay 1:   Today Was a Good Day
    Essay 2:   Is Your Life's Work a Calling?
              Lessons from Global Neurosurgery
    Essay 3:   Selflessness and Selfishness
    Essay 4:   Mismatched Expectations
    Essay 5:   Curiosity and Listening
    Essay 6:   Boundaries
    Essay 7:   On Being Judgmental
    Essay 8:   To Teach Is to Give
    Essay 9:   Doctor, Do Not Abandon Your Patient
    Essay 10: Suffering
    Essay 11: Facing Rejection
    Essay 12: Emotional Health in the Midst of the Covid-19 Pandemic
    Essay 13: Mindfulness
    Essay 14: Thank You, Dr. Xue
    Essay 15: Empowerment
    Essay 16: The Imposter Syndrome
    Essay 17: Hello, How Are You?
    Essay 18: The Dunning Krueger Effect
    Essay 19: Today Will Be a Good Day
    Essay 20   Opportunity

SECTION THREE: INTRODUCTION
LESSONS FROM THE MEDICAL ARENA 87

    Essay 1:   Bias, Therapeutic Illusion and the Illusion of Control
    Essay 2:   Managing Illness
    Essay 3:   The Art of Surgery
    Essay 4:   Process vs. Conclusion-Based Research
              Why Should We Care?

Essay 5:	Who Is Driving the Bus?	
Essay 6:	Pseudo-concordance and the Elephant in the Room	
Essay 7:	Doctor, I Trust You	
Essay 8:	Thank You	
Essay 9:	I'm Sorry	
Essay 10:	The Breakpoint	
Essay 11:	Dogma, Cost, and Healthcare	
Essay 12:	Clinical Equipoise	
Essay 13:	Fulfillment and Meaning	
Essay 14:	Highs and Lows	
Essay 15:	What the Pandemic Has Taught Us	
Essay 16:	Defining Limiters	
Essay 17:	Less Can Be More	
Essay 18:	The Good Old Days	
Essay 19:	Comparison Is the Thief of Joy	

SECTION FOUR: INTRODUCTION
SOCIETAL ISSUES AND OBLIGATIONS 135

Essay 1:	The International Patient Experience: A "World" of Difference	
Essay 2:	Hate: A Worldwide Conundrum	
Essay 3:	Black Lives Matter	
Essay 4:	On Being Vulnerable	
Essay 5:	Right versus Privilege	

Acknowlegments 149

Praises for *Today Was a Good Day* 150

FOREWORD

Neurosurgeons hold enormous responsibility in their skilled but mortal hands. They can help repair and restore health, vigor, and movement. They can animate human life. Unless, of course, sometimes they just can't. I'd call the responsibilities of a neurosurgeon are almost paralyzing, except, of course, that's no way to operate.

In *Today Was a Good Day: A Collection of Essays from the Heart of a Neurosurgeon*, Dr. Edward Benzel distills decades of wisdom he's acquired from the matchless experience of helping patients, staff, and neurosurgeons face and fulfill their enormous responsibilities—and get better in all ways.

I have the good fortune (and I really do consider it that) to have been in Dr. Benzel's care at Cleveland Clinic. He has always treated me and my family with care, concern, and compassion. My only complaint (and really, I'm reconciled to it) is that he apparently implanted a chip in my spine during surgeries that turned me into a Cleveland Cavaliers fan. Each time I've awakened in the recovery room, a staffer gently inquired, "How are you? How are you?" And I've replied, thanks to Dr. B's surgical mastery, "Don't worry about me. How's LeBron?" I'll have to have that looked at some day.

It is impressive to read this collection of essays and appreciate how many times this celebrated neurosurgeon and educator urges his colleagues to evince empathy and even humility. This might upset our view of head-strong surgeons, venerated at the top of their profession. But Ed Benzel insists that medical professionals at all levels understand that the relationship between doctor and patient, surgeon and patient, is a partnership. The surgeon needs their patient to describe not only how they feel, but what they may fear. The patient needs the surgeon to not only be empathetic, but show it, in detailed ways, so that patients will feel confident to entrust their care to someone whom they feel shares their concerns and respects them. His advice is both elevated and practical.

And Dr. Benzel presents this insightful and valuable book at a time when the world is cautiously sticking it's head out from under the shell of the Covid-pandemic. We will all have our stories: the friends and families we missed (and, too often, lost), the hopes fractured, opportunities lost, and fears instilled. As Dr. Benzel notes, neurosurgeons in particular had the unaccustomed sensation of feeling somehow less useful and essential than medical professionals who could address the overwhelming threat of the pandemic. Guilt was a human response. Many felt they had spent so much of their lives preparing themselves to be useful. Quite suddenly, their usefulness seemed diminished.

But Dr. Benzel reminds us that we all discovered sources of resilience during the pandemic, on which we might call on, in unexpected ways, is the future.

Ed Benzel has written a book from the heart of a great neurosurgeon. But of course the wisdom he has been able to acquire through opening his heart to so many patients can remind all of us, whatever we do, to be open to and humble for one another, and to make time to recharge ourselves with time and love. The professional skills of a neurosurgeon cannot be delivered to their patients, or survive, without human skills, too. The lessons Dr. Benzel offers, to neurosurgeons and those of us who turn to them for help and understanding, can shine a light out for us all.

—Scott Simon, *broadcaster and author*

PREFACE

It was November 12, 2010, that I received an email from one of my partners, Tom Mroz. We are both spine surgeons at the Cleveland Clinic. Tom is an orthopedic surgeon, about two decades younger than me, and I a neurosurgeon. I had sent him a piece I wrote. To be honest with you, I cannot remember the paper or topic, but it evidently had an impact on Tom, as illustrated by his email to me:

> Ed:
>
> I just finished reading your paper, it's great and supports my assertion—you should write a book.
>
> When I was in Memphis sitting in clinic with Kevin (a neurosurgeon and spine surgeon), he told me something that was forever etched on my mind: "Every neurosurgeon has his own personal cemetery" (and lives with it for the rest of his life). I knew that was a bit much for me; I didn't want that kind of responsibility.
>
> An elaboration on my assertion: Neurosurgeons represent less than 0.1% of the population, and among the lay population neurosurgery is perhaps the most intriguing specialty in medicine—an area where so much is left unknown, and yet is so inescapably a part of every person's life (i.e., emotions, memory, etc.). You have had a long career with more experiences in the clinical arena than any of us know of. You have a unique ability to think outside the box and to communicate that to many different people, and *you're a chairman of one of the best neurosurgery programs and best hospitals in the world, and one of the most well-known neurosurgeons in the world*. Further, most people don't run their age in miles on their birthday. Perhaps you

do it to define your limits, and perhaps it's no one's business why you do it. But it's interesting. People would be fascinated, and perhaps inspired.

My view of the book: The book should not be written for physicians. It should be written for people. It should provide a view into a neurosurgeon's career, complete with professional and personal triumphs, and motivational, challenging and life-changing moments. It allows the reader to actually experience the weight of critical moments that a neurosurgeon himself/herself experiences—the losses, the happiness, the sadness, the high blood pressure, the anxiety, the tachycardia. How does a neurosurgeon evolve over time with each of these extreme experiences? How does it shape him/her, in this case, you? It should give the readership an understanding of the "mind," of what memory and emotion are—if written well, this will grab people. All of this is woven into your life—your philosophies, your limits, what it takes to succeed, what it takes to lead, how people can fail. It's about "life" as much as it is about neurosurgery. It's your statement.

Remember, success in movies, music, books, plays and the like is in very large part predicated on empathy. It moves the recipient. I'm not saying write a book for money or more prestige but write one to move the masses in some way. It would be an extraordinary gift.

Just a thought,
Tom

For the "what it's worth column," the institution Tom is referring to is the Cleveland Clinic. I was the chairman of neurosurgery for ten years, from 2007–2017, and am now an Emeritus Chairman of Neurosurgery. Running my age in miles on my birthday refers to me running my age in miles at some time, approximating my birthday from age 40 to age 64 (I am now 74, as this book is taking form). I stopped "running my age" at age 64 because I became slower as the distances became longer. Something had to give.

I had yearned to write a book such as this for years, no, decades. To be clear, I have written many books, but they were medical books, predominantly spine related. To the vast majority of people, they would be extraordinarily boring and of little utility.

Regardless, I tucked Tom's email neatly in a file on my computer and it stayed in the file untouched for over a decade. In the meantime, I had become Editor-in-Chief of *World Neurosurgery*, an international neurosurgery monthly journal, in 2015. It was in this role that I began writing monthly Editor-in-Chief letters. At first they were mostly associated with "housekeeping" issues, pertaining mostly to mission statements, new sections, and the like. In and around 2018, I began addressing issues such as empathy, communication, resilience, Black Lives Matter, and other topics that pertain to how we (and this case, specifically neurosurgeons) carry out our lives and the effect on quality of life. Upon rereading Tom's email, the notion of restating and recrafting these messages for all people, not just neurosurgeons, might be of value to some—and, as such, the wheels began to churn faster regarding how I might accomplish this, even if only of value to a few.

So, I began categorizing the relevant Editor-in-Chief letters into topically related groupings. I provide the original letter that was written for neurosurgeons, and modified for lay public consumption, in each essay. Chapters are grouped into sections. I fully recognize that the grouping strategy is nebulous, but at least it represents an attempt at achieving order. Of note in this regard, most of the chapters are inserted in order of publication in *World Neurosurgery*. In each essay I translate for the lay reader and draw on my life experiences to drive home points and hopefully add clarity.

In this book, I "bob and weave" by liberally employing segues when the moment seemed appropriate to me. This may be confusing to some. If so, I apologize.

In the end, as suggested by Tom, this work will hopefully be perceived as a gift that might move the masses, even if the "masses" are small.

Who would have thought that I would be writing the book, as Tom suggested? My ultimate intent was and is to provide some insights into leadership, effective communication and fulfillment from the perspective of a neurosurgeon—from the heart and soul of a neurosurgeon. I hope to accomplish this, in a way, by translating what is important to neurosurgeons into a format that makes it relevant to all humans.

In a sense, this book is a collection of essays by me, for you. They represent my "take" on each subject. Each essay can stand alone, but taken as a collective they theoretically provide much greater meaning and, hence, impact. Of note, there exists a randomness regarding the order of the essays. This is somewhat by design, since each essay/essay is, indeed, a stand-alone piece. They are somewhat categorized into four sections. As a humorous closure to this preface, when I had my wife Mary read Tom's email she commented and I, in turn, shared with Tom: Mary says that really famous people (like ex-presidents) write leadership books—not schmucks like me. (The word "schmuck" was likely my translation of what she actually said.)

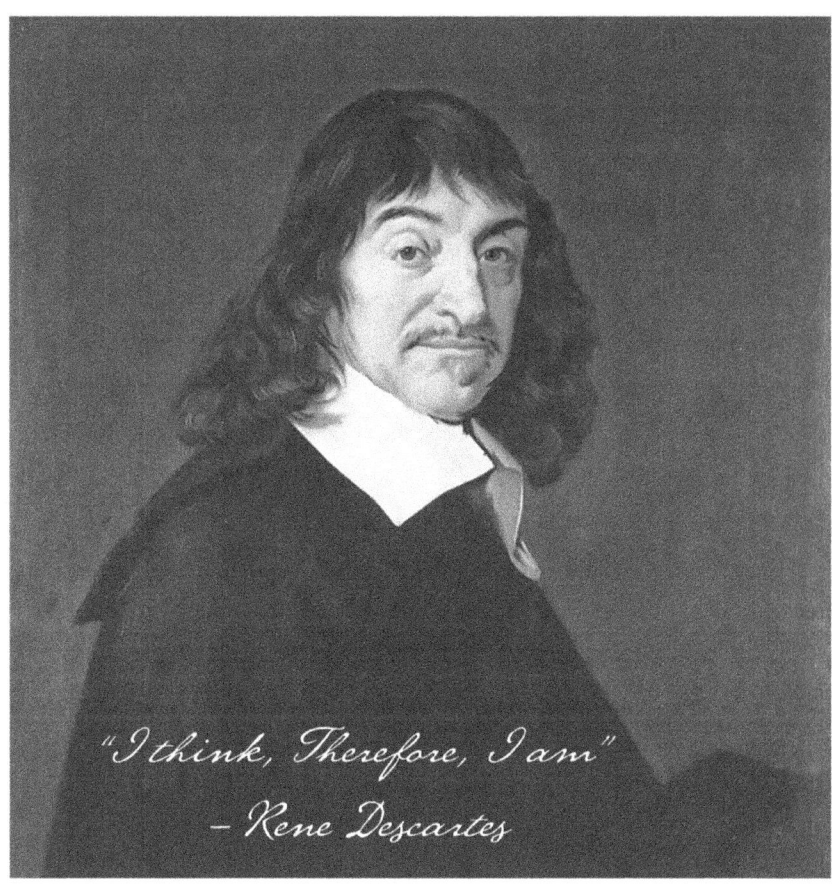

SECTION ONE: INTRODUCTION

*I Think, Therefore, I Am:
Crafting a Better Version of Ourselves*
....

"I think, therefore, I am" was penned by René Descartes (1596 – 1650). He was a French-born philosopher, mathematician, and scientist. He spent a large portion of his working life in the Dutch Republic, initially serving the Dutch States Army of Maurice of Nassau, Prince of Orange and the Stadtholder of the United Provinces.

Section One

His statement "I think, therefore, I am" probes, almost mystically, into the depths of what constitutes who we are and the "meaning of life."

Tom Mroz, an orthopedic spine surgeon partner of mine (also referenced in the Preface of this book), and I have had a decade-long dialogue regarding "the meaning of life" (for lack of a better term). He has been petitioning me to write a book. He states in a recent email, "People are intrigued with the workings of the brain. People are intrigued by the mind and brain; what motivates, what remembers, where does hope come from, how do we adapt, why can't we forget some things, where does consciousness come from. Part of the intrigue for people stems from wondering about life and our own mortality, our place in life, and of one's future (if there is one) beyond life. At what point does the mind stop and soul (if you believe in one) begin. Or, are they one 'thing.' Anyone aware of their own existence and their own mortality would be interested in such a book."

Mind you, I am not a philosopher. I, however, am intrigued, as was Tom Mroz, regarding the proof of our existence and what defines Tom Mroz, Ed Benzel, and all the rest of us. In the pages that follow in this section, I address many topics that pertain to how neurosurgeons interact with others and how each of us can use introspection to modify who we are—using tools and strategies such as empathy, respect, stress management, and much, much more. By thinking about these topics, we put ourselves in a position to shape our mind and thus shape who we are. We can become a better person via this process. I emphasize that there is no ceiling here. There is always room for improvement.

In this regard, Descartes' statement "I think, therefore I am" takes on a new meaning as we self-examine, as individuals, via thinking and then shaping who we are ("I am"). Tom's questions are very poignant and, at the same time, elusive. We can shape who we are to some extent, but we cannot answer Tom's existential questions, i.e., "what motivates, what remembers, where does hope come from, how do we adapt, why can't we forget some things, where does consciousness come from?"

What we can do is to make self-improvement one of our highest priorities. We can work on becoming more empathic, more respectful of others, striking an appropriate balance between selflessness and selfishness, becoming more curious and more

Section One

cognizant of our boundaries as well as those of others, being nonjudgmental, and becoming trustworthy and more mindful.

Each of us has the skillset to establish who we are ("I am") via thinking and then, in turn, shaping our mind, with the goal of becoming a better person. The message for us all—keep thinking and strive to make who we are a better version of ourselves than the prior version.

This process fundamentally comes down to empathy, respect, adapting to and modifying our responses to stress and, finally, leadership. The boundaries between these are blurry, though. Empathy, indeed, is foundational and leadership is overarching. The interplay between them results in a "dance" of sorts within each of us as we struggle to lead empathically. Respect for others is imperative. Successfully adapting to and modifying stress allows us to effectively choreograph the "dance" between the integral parts of each component—empathy, respect, and leadership.

Finally, many topics are addressed in multiple chapters. Please do not interpret this as redundancy. Rather, understand that we as adults have increasingly shorter attention spans as we age. Repetition is a way of conveying critical and vital information and principles in such a way that they are remember. My view here, "repetition is good."

Section One

Essay 1
Empathy: A Foundational Attribute

Arguably, empathy is the most important communication tool that we humans have at our disposal. My wife Mary, my best friend, part-time proofreader and sounding board, points out that "empathy" is a nebulous term. As such, discussions pertaining to empathy are similarly nebulous. Regardless, here goes.

Rarely do any of us wake up in the morning with the goal of causing conflict in the course of conversations with family, colleagues or acquaintances, though all of us, even the most angelic of us, occasionally do. All of us care. We care about relationships. We want our conversations to be productive and collegial. So why then do we end up in conversational conflict when such is rarely our intention?

Caring, evidently, is not enough. What, then, is missing? What is missing is the "expression of the fact that we care." What do I mean by this? All we need to do is express the fact that we care. PERPETUALLY expressing the fact that we care should be our goal with all of our interpersonal communications and interactions. We must aggressively strive to NEVER let our guard down during moments of lapsed self-awareness. ALL OF US can do better here. We can, indeed, improve social-awareness skills, and hence our expression of caring, but in order to do such we must work at it. We must endeavor to constantly be more "self-aware" and perpetually strive to express the fact that we care.

"Moments of lapsed self-awareness" is the operative phrase here. Self-awareness is also a nebulous entity that is difficult to define (an awareness of one's own personality or individuality) and even more difficult to operationalize. Being aware of oneself and how we project ourselves in conversation is a truly difficult task. Self-awareness is integrally interwoven with social-awareness (the ability to comprehend and appropriately react to both broad problems of society and interpersonal struggles). These terms can be thought of in the context of how we project ourselves, versus how we perceive and respond to the needs of others.

Section One

More often than not, we have a good grasp of our own self-awareness. But "moments of lapsed self-awareness" can often rear its ugly head, as conversations shift from collegial interactions to interactions in which discord and conflict emerge. Such shifts are occasionally inevitable, but most are preventable.

We either care or we don't. If one does not care, adverse interpersonal relationships cannot be addressed. I surmise that that the vast majority of those who will read this book care about relationships or they would not be in their current, often "revered" position as respected citizens and scholars. Empathy, however, embodies much more than caring. As previously stated, we must perpetually seek to express the fact that we care. This requires a focus on self-awareness. We should strive to heighten our self-surveillance regarding our actions and conversations by focusing on caring and letting others know it. Most importantly, we should strive to eliminate "moments of lapsed self-awareness." Such is not easy. If it were, the world would be a much better place than it is today.

Section One

Essay 2

Respect

"R-E-S-P-E-C-T, find out what it means to me."
– Aretha Franklin

With the passing of Aretha Franklin (1942–2018), the world lost an iconic singer, songwriter, civil rights activist, actress, and pianist. The Queen of Soul's words regarding respect reverberate through many of our brains as we ponder the state of our own respect and the respect due others. Conveying respect and, in turn, being respected is an integral component of communication and, in fact, fulfillment.

Respect is a two-way street. It is difficult to respect an individual who does not respect others, including you. So, how does one convey respect? Well, for starters, one should be *in the moment* during conversations with others. Focus on the person and their words. Express concern, be empathic, and *listen*. Communicate via meaningful dialogue and avoid monologue. Both the conveyance of respect and meaningful conversations are, indeed, two-way streets. Empathy rules here; both caring and expressing the fact that you care are an unbeatable duo.

Having a meaningful conversation with another requires the establishment of mutual respect, usually via the creation of an emotional connection. The latter is nurtured by developing lines of communication that are based on a genuine interest in each other, with the mutual goal of a shared commitment to something. In a doctor-patient relationship, a shared commitment to health is a conduit through which communication lines pass and through which respect may be conveyed via the two-way street. Another example is a shared commitment to success of a work-related project. With both, the communicators are creating an emotional connection by mutually striving for success. The process is facilitated by the expression of mutual respect.

What may be more important here is the consideration of what to not do. Don't attend to emails on your cell phone during conversations; rather, attend to the other

Section One

parties in the conversation. Be "in the moment" with them. Don't alter discussion flow for your own purpose; rather, convey the fact that you are listening—truly listening. Communicate via a dialogue, not a monologue. Don't disregard events and situations that are important to others in the conversation; rather, express interest in your friend's granddaughter's wedding or her new house.

It's the little things that make a difference here. The demonstration of respect is all about being a human being who is genuinely concerned about another human being. What it is not is the seeking of respect by way of a *demand (demanding respect)*. It simply does not work that way. True respect is earned by paying attention to the little things. It is in this way, and this way only, that we can legitimately *command respect*.

The words from Aretha Franklin "R-E-S-P-E-C-T, find out what it means to me" have a special meaning when taken in the context of the aforementioned. Respect is important to all humans. Respecting people for who they are, the good they do, and what they bring to the table means a lot to them. When we humans feel respected, we tend to respond in kind.

Sometimes, though, we forget to convey respect, particularly when we let our guard down. Let us all seek to raise the conveyance of respect for others to the top of our conscience and make it a communication priority. The world will then become a better place. It's just like empathy. It is not enough to care. We must express the fact that we care.

Section One

Essay 3
Stress and Stress Recovery

"Keep close to nature's heart… and break clear away once in a while, and climb a mountain or spend a week in the woods. Wash your spirit clean."

– John Muir

There exists research that indicates that sleep is critical for achieving longevity (not too much and not too little sleep). I was impressed by the finding that suboptimal sleep during the work week can be compensated by "sleeping in" on weekends (.*https://www.marketwatch.com/story/theres-one-critical-reason-you-should-sleep-in-this-weekend-2018-05-25* This is interesting, since many people are driven, driven in a way that causes their "motor" to rarely slow down or to take a break. This subjects "the driven" to the risk of succumbing to the ravages of stress and the toll that stress takes on the body and mind of active, driven, and seemingly tireless people. To sleep more, if only on weekends, may be a key to stress reduction or, perhaps more appropriately stated, stress recovery.

James Loehr is a sports psychologist and author. I read one of his works years ago, and found it to be very interesting. This book, *Stress for Success,* was of great interest to me, as it presented a somewhat counterintuitive concept. In his book, Loehr comments on a common misconception regarding stress—i.e., that it should be avoided or, at the very least, minimized. We commonly deal with stress via an avoidance strategy. It turns out, though, that avoiding certain stressors may be detrimental to skill acquisition and development.

Let's think this through. If an individual's desire is to become increasingly more accomplished at his/her craft over time and to develop the skills necessary to effectively manage increasingly complex problems, he/she must expose him/herself to a series of situations where the exposure to stress is progressively escalated. The more the individual is exposed to increasing levels of stress, the greater his/her ability to manage such and, in a sense, the more accomplished he/she becomes.

Section One

Looking at this concept from another perspective, the long-distance runner did not develop the endurance to run a marathon by avoiding stress—i.e., the stress associated with intervals of increased distances and increased speed. The act of acquiring endurance is stressful. Such involves the progressive exposure to ever-increasing amounts of physical and mental challenges (stress).

Those who are "driven" to succeed in business, long-distance running and life in general, hence, have a common means to achieve an end—i.e., progressively escalating exposure to stress. If such is so, how can we rationalize the management of stress via its avoidance? In reality, for the most part we can't. Yes, we should avoid unnecessary or pathological stressors, such as non-productive conflict and discourse. We, however, should separate the latter from the stress that causes us to become better at what we do. This includes becoming a better person, and a more productive and fulfilled individual.

As Loehr points out, the answer is simple—we need to intermittently and repetitively recover from stress; i.e., "stress recovery." What a concept. So, John Muir's aforementioned reference to the importance of breaking away to the mountain or to the woods to "wash your spirit clean" suggests that such divergences from the stress associated with daily life is vital. This stress recovery mechanism restores inner peace and calm. Similarly, the notion of getting home from work at a reasonable time and taking a "several-hour mini-vacation with family" in the evening before bed, and without the distractions of work, diverges significantly from the stresses experienced at work. As mentioned, recent research indicates, people who "sleep in" on weekends live longer.[1] "Sleeping in" on weekends diverges from the daily weekday life routine. In a way, it represents a component of a vacation.

We have enough stress in our lives, but at the same time we must always strive to become better at what we do. We can only do this through exposure to stress. So, we should continue to expose ourselves to the stressors that make us better and stronger. More importantly, however, we must craft and protect the access to those activities or inactivates that allow us to recover from stress. Take mini-vacations. Recharge. "Wash your spirit clean." It appears that we will live longer, be healthier and become even better humans if we do.

Section One

Essay 4

Leadership

Leadership is the overarching umbrella over communication that contains, beneath it, all the essential components that will be discussed in Section 2 of this book. Let us start with a definition that we can embrace with ease: "Leadership is the art of causing others to deliberately create a result that otherwise would not have happened." Simple enough. What follows here is my "take" on leadership and how this pertains to each and every one of us.

We are all leaders! But, what defines a leader? I will begin by discussing and characterizing the attributes of effective leaders. Leaders are selfless. They give to others. I was particularly "taken" by a segment of the book *When Breath Becomes Air* by Paul Kalanithi, which I also reference in Section 2, Essay 2. It is so impactful that I reference it here and in Section 2, Essay 2. Paul Kalanithi was a neurosurgery trainee at Stanford who died of cancer. During his last years, he wrote one of the most compelling reads that have passed by my eyes. The segment I reference here occurred during his medical school years at Stanford. A group of students wished to alter their student mission statement by eliminating language that referred to physicians being selfless and giving to their patients their all. His commentary on this is very revealing: "…several students argued for the removal of the language insisting we place our patients' interests above our own. The rest of us didn't allow this discussion to continue for long. The words stayed. This kind of egotism struck me as antithetical to medicine and, it should be noted, entirely reasonable. Indeed, this is how 99 percent of people select their jobs: pay, work environment, hours. But that's the point. Putting lifestyle first is how you find a job—not a calling."

A job, in a sense, is a means to an end, e.g., salary for sustenance. However, in a way, it could be a calling as well. For example, it may provide the wherewithal to support and nurture a family. This, in turn, provides an intangible value to the family, to the community and, in the end, the world. Looking at it this way may cause us to "see" many jobs as callings.

Section One

How we view our life's work is critical. Do we view it as a job or a calling? And, if we view it as a job, should we rethink our position on this subject and in life? I will not belabor this point here, but such is worthy for all of us to contemplate. Regardless, I make the case that all of us, as the leaders we are, should be selfless when it comes down to interactions with others, specifically those who we are able to help.

On the other side of the coin, leaders should also be selfish. They must be protective of time with family and their own wellbeing. What all of us must do as leaders, and I again emphasize that we are all leaders, is strike a balance between selflessness and selfishness.

Leaders have passion for what they do. Their work is not just a job; it represents, or at least it should be representative of, a fire in our belly regarding purpose and meaning for our life's work. If we can make this so, we will have transformed our job into a calling.

Leaders are egalitarian—i.e., of, relating to, or believing in the principle that all people are equal and deserve equal rights and opportunities. Leaders must never play favorites and must always treat those whom we lead with utmost respect. Remember, I am not pointing at some and not others here. All of us who chose to lead are leaders.

Leaders should be socially aware. They must be aware of their environment. In so doing, they must be perpetually empathic by focusing on expressing the fact that they care. Leaders must have a vision and develop strategies to achieve goals. Leaders must have self-direction skills by exhibiting the ability to make decisions and solve problems. Leaders must harbor the ability to motivate others to create results that otherwise would not have happened. Finally, leaders must be self-aware: "How am I coming across in this conversation? This can only be achieved by listening and, specifically, by listening reflectively. For example, if one is asked "How are you?" one should listen for the response and act accordingly.

Theodore Roosevelt stated: "People ask the difference between a leader and a boss. The leader leads and the boss drives." Lead! Don't drive! In this vein, there exist many types or categories of leadership—including transactional, autocratic, laissez-fair, democratic, bureaucratic, leadership, charismatic, managerial, operational,

Section One

transformational, thought and servant leadership. All but the last two are based on reward and punishment.

Thought leaders are individuals who are recognized as an authority in a field and whose expertise is sought and often rewarded. We all seek to be knowledgeable and sought after for that knowledge. Servant leaders serve the people they lead. This implies that employees are an end in and of themselves, rather than a means to an organizational goal or purpose. Servant leaders genuinely lead by enhancing the effectiveness of the people they lead.

Leaders work. They work hard at being a leader. Leadership is not easy—not easy at all. Leaders are also competent. Competence, in its ultimate form, requires perpetual assessment and reassessment. Leaders perpetually reflect. Finally, leaders are wise. They make decisions that are based on fact and not on self-promotion or gain. Bottom line, great leaders do what's right! So, the take-home message here is presented in the form of a recommendation: Lead!!! At the end of the day, strive to feel like clicking your heels on your way home. If you feel this way, you know it was a good day.

Section One

Essay 5
Fatigue, or Is It Burnout?

Definitions:
Fatigue: extreme tiredness resulting from mental or physical exertion or illness.
Burnout: a state of emotional, physical, and mental exhaustion caused by excessive and prolonged stress.

This essay should be taken in the context of having been written in the midst of the COVID-19 pandemic. At the time of reading, the COVID scene will most certainly have changed.

"I am really stressed and drained. Is this fatigue or is it burnout?" "I struggle with routine duties." "I cannot shake the burden of a complication. The toll of the complication seems much greater than in days gone by." These are paraphrased utterances of some of my surgical colleagues. To answer the first question, I see COVID-related fatigue as one of the symptoms that fall under the overarching umbrella of burnout. Things move slowly and work-related duties mount. For many, this scenario becomes suffocating—leading to depression and outright burnout. This is seemingly an "unshakeable" condition that, to one degree or another, affects us all.

Perhaps one of the most poignant comments, however, came as a commentary from a younger partner regarding the opportunity to escape the stresses of our current COVID and political environment. Of note, I am in my 70s, and nearly two decades his senior. In a moment of frustration, likely resulting from fatigue and burnout, he stated to me, "Ed, you are so lucky. You can leave this mess (i.e., retire), should you choose to. I cannot."

I have never thought of being "old" as an advantage. In many respects, though, in the current COVID and stressful medical environment, it may in fact be. I continue to work as a neurosurgeon because I love it. I love the patients. I love the students,

Section One

residents, fellows and all the supporting cast of people who are essential parts of the healthcare team. I love to teach. I love my partners. I love my job as Editor-in-Chief of *World Neurosurgery*. **BUT**, I possess an advantage that affords me the opportunity to dodge the "other side" of work—the increasing complexity of the clinical care environment, complications, the COVID-related isolation, the incredible yet veiled stress associated with the unknown, and on and on. Yes, I can afford to retire, essentially whenever I feel compelled to do such.

Regarding the unknown, I guess that at my age I am at a greater risk from COVID than others who are decades younger. In March, April and May 2020 the COVID-related risk seemed great. I worked virtually from home during much of this early phase. During this phase, 19 (and quite possibly more) neurosurgeons worldwide succumbed to COVID-19 (their names were listed on the December 2020) issue cover of *World Neurosurgery*). Most were over sixty years of age.

Months later, though, we became complacent. The concerns of months prior seem to be trivialized—at least on the surface. Now we expose ourselves to an even greater risk—and internalize our feelings regarding risk. This all takes place in front of a backdrop of isolation. This results in COVID-related fatigue and burnout.

The mounting stresses, and the resultant fatigue and burnout, cause all of us, neurosurgeons and non-neurosurgeons alike, to take pause and think through each of our individual strategies for the future. Those who are far from retirement must approach workplace career-related decisions very differently from those who are at or near retirement age.

So, how do each of us as individuals manage fatigue and burnout? James Loehr, in his book *Stress for Success*, emphasizes the importance of seeking stress in order to become stronger and more resilient. However, as emphasized by Loehr and expounded upon by me in Essay 3 in this section, we must recover from stress. We cannot omit the second part of this two-part recipe for success—i.e., stress recovery. Continued exposure to relentless stress results in fatigue and burnout. Stress recovery in the form of vacations, stress-free weekends and evenings, exercise, etc.—during which we discuss, think and act on things not work related. We must separate our work-related stress, and social/political stress for that matter, from our stress recovery strategy. We

Section One

must strive to seek a balance between stress and obligatory stress recovery. As a final note, and in the spirit of transparency, I am personally working on achieving this balance. I must admit, I am not there yet—not even close.

Section One

Essay 6

Competence

I ask that the reader, physicians as well as lay people, sit back and think how the following scenario applies to you. We will focus here, though, on the growth of a neurosurgeon. Everyone else can create their own scenario, based their profession and professional growth..

As an exercise, I would like to hypothetically take a neurosurgeon back to medical school in order to reflect on the neurosurgeon's journey through time as he/she gradually acquires skills and knowledge; i.e., competence. As a medical student, the future neurosurgeon, relatively speaking, did not know much and did not really know how much he/she did not know. The future neurosurgeon was essentially *unconsciously incompetent*. Such unconscious incompetence is the rule, rather than the exception, for all of us as we transition onto a path towards a career.

Oh, but wait—there is more. As the future neurosurgeon approached the internship year (the first year after medical school), he/she began to realize that he/she knew very little, in the big scheme of things, and that the amount of requisite information that was to be gathered, distilled and assimilated was daunting—and downright frightening. At the moment of this realization, the future neurosurgeon transitioned from *unconscious incompetence* to *conscious incompetence*. Knowing how much you do not know can indeed be suffocating. These are very unsettling times for a young physician or for anyone in a similar or analogous situation.

As the early years of residency training passed by, the neurosurgery resident (future neurosurgeon in training) acquired a massive foundation of knowledge and a trove of skills. The future neurosurgeon honed in on knowledge acquisition. In fact, he/she became a quick learner by working at it—really working at it. The work seemed, at times, to be excessive and never ending, but the future neurosurgeon prevailed. As such, he/she successfully transitioned into the next phase of learning and overall competence—termed *conscious competence*. During this phase, the future neu-

Section One

rosurgeon and others in their respective scenarios needed to continuously study and work for every morsel of knowledge that one could gobble up.

As the neurosurgeon in training approached the chief year (last year of training) and into early practice, he/she began to make decisions and act reflexively and with less effort. As part of this reflexive process, habits were formed. Clinical decisions and the act of surgery became "second nature." As the neurosurgeon entered this phase of competence, he/she harbored a sense of confidence—a confidence that may or may not be appropriate or justified. This phase is termed *unconscious competence*. The reason that the confidence acquired may or not be appropriate or justified is related to the habitual nature of the actions performed during this phase. To clarify, there are two types of habits—good and bad habits. If any of us act reflexively with our actions based on bad habits, suboptimal outcomes may often ensue.

So, how do we deal with the tendency to rely on habits? Perhaps the best strategy is to continuously reflect on our thought process, our actions and our results. This, the ultimate phase of competence, is termed *reflective competence*.

The words of Sir William Osler (a very famous physician), in his 1905 treatise, *The Student Life,* resonates here. "Begin early to make a threefold category—*clear cases, doubtful cases, mistakes*. And learn to play the game fair. No self-deception. No shrinking from the truth. Mercy and consideration for the other man. But none for yourself, upon whom you have to keep an incessant watch…. It is only by getting your cases grouped in this way that you can make any real progress in your (continuing) education; only in this way can you gain wisdom from experience." Harvey Cushing (in a sense, the grandfather of neurosurgery) applied these principles meticulously. He recorded, photographed, drew, and documented the details of his operations—so that he could reflect on prior experiences in order to optimize future actions. If each of us, regardless of our profession, achieve such a level of self-reflection, we will have become *reflectively competent*. We all have a long way to go here, but it is not too late to begin or accelerate the process. Let's all begin by increasing our focus on reflection and honest self-assessment—followed by action based on our reflections.

Section One

Essay 7
The Humility Button

Humility (Merriam-Webster definition):
Freedom from pride or arrogance. The quality or state of being humble.

Humble (Merriam-Webster definition):
Reflecting, expressing, or offered in a spirit of deference or submission.
Ranking low in a hierarchy or scale. Insignificant. Unpretentious.

"In 1941, Sergeant James Allen Ward was awarded the Victoria Cross for climbing out onto the wing of his Wellington bomber at thirteen thousand feet to extinguish a fire in the starboard engine. Secured only by a rope around his waist, he smothered the fire and returned along the wing to the aircraft's cabin. Winston Churchill, an admirer of swashbuckling exploits, summoned the shy New Zealander to 10 Downing Street. Struck dumb with awe in Churchill's presence, Ward was unable to answer the prime minister's questions. Churchill surveyed the unhappy hero with some compassion. 'You must feel very humble and awkward in my presence,' he said.

"'Yes, sir,' managed Ward.

"'Then you can imagine how humble and awkward I feel in yours,' said Churchill."

Being humble, truly humble, is rarely achieved in its purest form. A perusal of the definitions of humility and humble may leave one confused. What, in fact, is true humility? Sergeant Ward exhibited uncontrollable reflexive and, hence, natural humility in the presence of Winston Churchill. Such may be considered true humility. Mr. Churchill in his conversation with Sergeant Ward, on the other hand, used his vulnerability as an admirer of Sergeant Ward's heroics to pay Sergeant Ward a compliment of the highest order. In so doing, Mr. Churchill used humility as a tool to even further honor a true hero.

My take on the definitions of humility and being humble involves genuinely placing oneself below others. Again, Sergeant Ward was unequivocally humble—

Section One

true/pure/naïve/beautifully innocent humility. He, in the presence of Mr. Churchill, put himself below practically all others in the hierarchal scheme of things. It wasn't about him (Sergeant Ward); it was about others, all others. And, Mr. Churchill, at least for a moment, put himself below others, as well, as he honored Sergeant Ward.

So, what can we learn from this interaction? Most of us are like Mr. Churchill. We try to be humble, but we have accomplished so much (in our own mind) and, in a sense, want the world to know of our accomplishments. Such a desire is not all that bad. We should be proud of our accomplishments. But, like Mr. Churchill, we should recognize when we need to push the "humility button" and show our vulnerabilities, in such a way that we honor others and put others above us as individuals. It is not about I, we, or us. It should truly and genuinely be about others. When we are humble, others come first. At least for that brief moment, for that brief moment Mr. Churchill lived in a world that was not about him. It, in fact, was about another—specifically Sergeant Ward.

Knowing when and how hard to push the "humility button" is a skill that few harbor. It involves the acquisition and application of social- self-awareness skillsets. We may or may not harbor these skills at a level that helps us effectively meander through the abyss of life, but these skills can be developed and nurtured. As we ponder thoughts like *How am I coming across?* or *What are others thinking about me?* we hone in on skills that help us become better communicators and provide the tools required to know when to and how hard to hit the "humility button." Bringing these and similar thoughts to the top of our consciousness will make us more effective communicators and perhaps a bit more humble. In the end, Winston Churchill, almost certainly unknowingly, provided us with a wonderful example of near perfect "humility button" employment. After all, humility is good. So, thank you, Sergeant Ward and Mr. Churchill, for teaching us a very important life lesson.

Section One

Essay 8

*Optimism versus Pessimism:
The Choice is Yours*

The COVID-19 pandemic era has caused significant stress worldwide. The stress related to fear of harm to self or loved ones at the hand of the virus, guilt regarding the perceived notion that one is not doing enough to help others during the pandemic, economic stressors, etc., was prevalent and ubiquitous during the early and middle phases of the pandemic.

A hidden and infrequently considered cause of stress is the uncertainty as to what the future holds. When will we have access to a vaccine (remember, this was written prior to the first year anniversary of the COVID-19 pandemic)? Will the vaccine be effective and durable? Will the vaccine, in fact, be safe? Will this isolation state ever end? Stress related to the fear of the unknown may be taking a much greater toll than commonly thought. Scott Litofsky, in his figure legend for the cover photo of the December 2020 issue of *World Neurosurgery* (a very compelling and intriguing work of art that was combined with the names of 19 neurosurgeons who, at that time, had succumbed to COVID-19), makes the following statement: *"While trying to maintain a positive attitude at work and to be an effective leader for my faculty, residents, and staff, I suppressed my own dark thoughts, only to have them emerge in this work. The release I felt while painting gave me the resilience to face the uncertain future."* Note, he emphasizes *resilience to face the uncertain future.*

The uncertainty of the future, in the face of so many losses, as shared in our memorials in *World Neurosurgery*, causes us to pause and reflect. The way in which we deal with the uncertainty can, in fact, diminish or escalate our stress levels.

One could choose to succumb or to prevail. Put another way, one could choose to be pessimistic or optimistic. The assumption of a negative posture regarding the COVID-19-related stressors creates an almost inevitable escalation of the already existing negativity-related stress. "Woe is me" essentially becomes the unspoken theme of such negativity. Allowing the fear of the unknown to dominate our lives is not healthy and

Section One

promotes and promulgates the negative and self-defeating nature of the process.

What if we all face the stressors of uncertainty in a positive way by remaining optimistic? If you were unable to rejoice in the graduation or a wedding of a loved one, or if you lost an opportunity to compete in a "once in a lifetime" event—you could address your lost opportunities by bemoaning such ("woe is me") or, alternatively, you could think positively by considering what you gave to humanity by way of your sacrifices. You minimized the risk of viral transmission by "staying home." You also have "grown" by virtue of the pandemic process. You have learned to become resilient. You have learned to utilize virtual communication advances (i.e., Zoom, Microsoft Team, etc.) to advance oftentimes more efficient and effective means of communication. You have learned that, after all, these alternative and effective means of communication can, in many ways, enhance both work-related and friends-and-family-related communication. One unequivocal and very notable advantage of this "forced isolation" is the remarkable increase in virtual webinars, seminars, and lectures, etc. This has, among many other things, provided much greater access to education for neurosurgeons and nearly all other professions in resource challenged middle- and low-income regions of the world. This alone should make all of us proud as we increase the dissemination of vital information worldwide.

Yes, we were stressed by not being able to see our loved ones during the pandemic. We were stressed by our losses. We were stressed by the uncertainty associated with "When will it end?" We are particularly stressed by the thought that the year of the unthinkable (2020) may linger far beyond the year of the unthinkable and perhaps become the decade of the unthinkable. However, by virtue of our resilience, we should accept our losses, as difficult as it may be, and face the future with optimism—knowing that we gave (sacrificed), some with their lives, so that we and others may live. Via an optimistic approach, we can grasp *"the resilience to face the uncertain future,"* in the words of Scott Litofsky. The pathway to resilience flows through optimism—NOT PESSIMISM!!! We must not cling to our memories of the "before," for it may never return just as it was. In looking forward, rather than backwards, we must live in the "now." We need to develop such a resilience motif so that we can meet further stressors like the pandemic with confidence and with optimism.

Section One

Essay 9
Self and Social Awareness

Self-awareness: an awareness of one's own personality or individuality

Social awareness: the ability to comprehend and appropriately react to both broad problems of society and interpersonal struggles

This essay embellishes upon Essay 1 in this section (Empathy) as the foundation for further discussion regarding self and social awareness. The topics of the two chapters are so intertwined that a clean separation is not possible. For starters, have you ever thought to yourself, *How am I coming across in this conversation?* If you have, and I suspect that all of us have on numerous occasions, you were exercising your self-awareness assessment skills. You wanted to determine if you were portraying yourself as you had intended. This is, indeed, a very difficult task. One never truly knows what others think of oneself. The best one can do is to keep the question at the forefront of consciousness and train to "read the field" more and more accurately. Repetitively practicing self-awareness skills leads to self-improvement and more and more effective communication.

Self awareness, in a sense, is a metric for assessing what others think or feel about us during real-life scenarios. Alternatively, social awareness is a de-facto metric for assessing one's ability to adapt to the societal (and social) challenges of life. With social-awareness, one assesses societal and social impact, whereas with self-awareness the metric assesses the impression or message that we convey to others during routine and not-so-routine conversations or via other forms of communication, such as email.

Armed with social-awareness skills, an individual may determine which of many responses may be the most socially appropriate response to a difficult question or social situation. The social-awareness skillset essentially uses a "social etiquette filter" that sorts out and discards inappropriate responses and allows only appropriate responses to pass through.

Section One

The entities social- and self-awareness are very different but are essentially inextricably linked. Asking oneself the question "How am I coming across?" and exercising the use of the "social etiquette filter" so that socially inappropriate responses are internalized and socially appropriate responses are externalized are frequently at play—working hand in hand to help us become more effective communicators and, in fact, more empathic communicators. As was discussed in Section 1, Essay 1 of this book, empathy is manifested by expressing the fact that we care. Although self awareness plays a predominant role in this (expressing the fact that we care), social awareness plays an accompanying synergistic role. This is much like the way that yin and yang complement each other. Social- and self-awareness skillsets address the task of expressing the fact that one cares from both poles of the task at hand—one by asking oneself "How am I coming across?" and the other by employing the "social etiquette filter" that separates the socially unacceptable from the acceptable. With practice, both can be developed and nurtured.

They say "Practice makes perfect." While perfection is rarely, if ever, achievable, it is both admirable and noble to seek such. Michelangelo's prayer, in a way, illustrates this point: "Lord, grant that I may always desire more than I can accomplish." Michelangelo perpetually sought perfection, but never quite achieved it, at least in his mind. If we could look at a personal goal of achieving excellent social and self awareness skills as if we were using Michelangelo's philosophy, we would become better communicators and more effective as leaders. We, indeed, can practice these skills. We simply need to put our mind to it by reminding ourselves to critically listen to what we say to others and to say to others what we truly want to convey. It's not difficult if we, indeed, put our minds to it!

Section One

Essay 10
Celebrate

Celebrate: to mark (something, such as an anniversary) by festivities or other deviations from routine
– Merriam-Webster

"Don't cry over spilled milk."
– Origin uncertain

"Necessity is the mother of invention."
– Origin uncertain

Celebrations take on multiple forms, with a near-infinite means to achieve a celebratory end. It seems, though, that we have had little to celebrate in these trying times of the COVID-19 pandemic era. We have had significant reason to mourn. We mourn the loss of lives at the hands of COVID-19, we reel in the financial devastation wrought by COVID-19, and we had meandered through the abyss of COVID-19 stressors that affected us all in ways we, as of yet, do not fully comprehend. As we emerge from the clutches in the pandemic, we also emerge from the shroud of prevailing uncertainty and fear of the unknown. Most of us have realized that, in fact, we do have much to celebrate.

However, we humans tend to dwell and perseverate on the past. We yearn for the time prior to an adverse event or outcome. The aphorism "Don't cry over spilled milk" should provide guidance to us as we gradually put the pandemic behind us and as we continue on our individual journeys through life. There is no point in dwelling on something that has already happened and, hence, cannot be changed. We tend to yearn for things to be like they were in the *"before"* (the time predating COVID-19). Alternatively, we should rather look forward and focus on what is in front of us (and not behind us). We need to work towards crafting a "new normal" that will hopefully be bigger and better than ever.

We might ask ourselves, what do we have to celebrate in these stressful COVID times? First and foremost, those of us reading this essay are alive. As such, we should have been, and should currently be, anticipating and preparing for a more positive future, a future where there is a global relaxation of social distancing and mask requirements—as well as the other changes that allow us to resume some semblance of normalcy worldwide. Such, alone, is worthy of celebration, but there is more.

What about the advances in communication, newfound time at home, and other unanticipated benefits that have "flowed" from the demands created by the COVID-19 pandemic? The aphorism "Necessity is the mother of invention" comes to mind here. We can and should also celebrate the world, with its governing bodies, decision makers and scientists coming together to develop and implement solutions such as safety guidelines, vaccines and the distribution of vaccines. We can and should celebrate the rapid development and deployment of virtual communication platforms. We can and should celebrate the global unity and sharing that evolved as a result of the pandemic. We can and should celebrate the emergence of the light at the end of the tunnel—and on and on.

Bottom line, we should celebrate and actively engage in the task of making this world an even better place in which to live. We can and should be proactive as we move forward, and not dwell on the tragedies that lay behind us. Of course, we should remain mindful of the financial hardships and of the human suffering that laid in the wake of the COVID-19 pandemic; however, we should keep in mind that remaining cognizant and mindful of the past is very different than "crying over spilled milk."

Section One

Essay 11
Experience

"Experience is what you get when you didn't get what you wanted."
– Randolph Frederick Pausch

Experience is the catalyst that transforms knowledge into wisdom. In a way, one could/should think of experience as the conduit between islands of knowledge by facilitating the bridging of knowledge gaps that separate the "islands of knowledge." As such, the "land mass" equivalent of wisdom grows and grows as we develop and mature—i.e., accumulate experience.

We "grow" by repetitively performing tasks. By doing such, we accumulate knowledge and develop habits, most of which are good habits. However, some of the developed habits are bad habits, which can lead to suboptimal results and adverse outcomes (also discussed in Essay 6 in this section). The mistakes, if recognized, can be rectified, thus paving the way towards modifying our own behavior by self-reflection—i.e., reflective competence.

Randolph Frederick Pausch, who was a professor of computer science, human–computer interaction, and design at Carnegie Mellon University in Pittsburgh, Pennsylvania, stated, "Experience is what you get when you didn't get what you wanted." This is very aptly put. "Not getting what you want" essentially correlates with the realization that an adverse event or a perceived suboptimal outcome occurred. When adverse events or suboptimal outcomes occur, we humans have two choices; we can either ignore the event, or we can rectify, if possible, and modify our behavior moving forward. We modify our behavior by connecting the dots, or "islands of knowledge," by acting on our own collective experiences.

It is interesting that we, indeed, can "learn from our mistakes." If we do not "see" our mistakes, though, we have lost a learning opportunity and lay the foundation for the development of bad habits. Bad habits can be very difficult to break, particularly if

Section One

they go unrecognized. Self-reflection is the key here. We must perpetually assess and reassess our actions and their results. We must perpetually reflect and self-scrutinize.

In the words of Sir William Osler, as appropriately presented in several chapters herein, in his treatise, *The Student Life,* 1905 (Dr. Osler is considered by most to be the father of what we now call Internal Medicine): "Begin early to make a threefold category—*clear cases, doubtful cases, mistakes*. And learn to play the game fair. No self-deception. No shrinking from the truth. Mercy and consideration for the other man. But none for yourself, upon whom you have to keep an incessant watch…. It is only by getting your cases grouped in this way that you can make any real progress in your (continuing) education; only in this way can you gain wisdom from experience." Although intended for physicians, Osler's comments apply to each and every one of us. Honest self-reflection is the key.

Section One

Essay 12
What the People of Ukraine Have Taught Us

"We must hang together gentlemen ... else we shall most assuredly hang separately."
– Benjamin Franklin,
a co-signer and editor of the United States Declaration of Independence

As the people of Ukraine and their president, Volodymyr Zelenskyy, take the world stage, a heartwarming and beautiful resolve emerges from the rubble, as the Ukraine people face death and destruction at the hands of a tyrant. The free world marvels at the courage, resilience, and commitment of these people. In Ukraine, the people are not polarized. They function as an innovative and committed unit. They "speak" with "one voice" and act with "one resolve." They are functioning in the absence of political self-interests overtly interfering with their mission.

I asked myself the question, would I and my fellow countrymen be as committed to our country (the United States) under similar circumstances? I think I would and many others would as well. I, however, worry that the politicization of things that should not be political, such as vaccinations, the provision of medical care, infrastructure spending, etc., in the United States, would bleed over into the decision-making process regarding a people's under-siege response to tyranny. The politicization tendency in the United States creates a polarization of the people. This does not appear to be an issue for the people of Ukraine.

So, what have the people of Ukraine taught us? My take on this is that they taught, and are currently teaching, us the importance of unity and the avoidance of polarizing divisiveness. The American Revolution serves as a similar example of a show of unity and resolve. Benjamin Franklin's statement to his fellow revolutionaries speaks volumes regarding the importance of unity: *"We must hang together gentlemen ... else we shall most assuredly hang separately."*

Section One

People become of one voice via compromise. Whether it be the American Revolution or Putin's War in Ukraine, "one voice" evolved because of compromise.

I see intense political strife in my country. Such strife threatens the fabric and foundation of the United States. The United States is not alone. Other countries suffer from similar polarizing politics as well. Compromise is the answer. Meeting in the middle and then speaking with one voice can become a tool for the achievement of success. This is what the people of Ukraine and, as an aside, the American Revolutionaries, taught us.

For me personally, I feel that I am in the middle of a game-changing life lesson. I am closely paying attention to my current teachers and mentors in this arena—the people of Ukraine. I thank them from the bottom of my heart for their courage and commitment via "one voice."

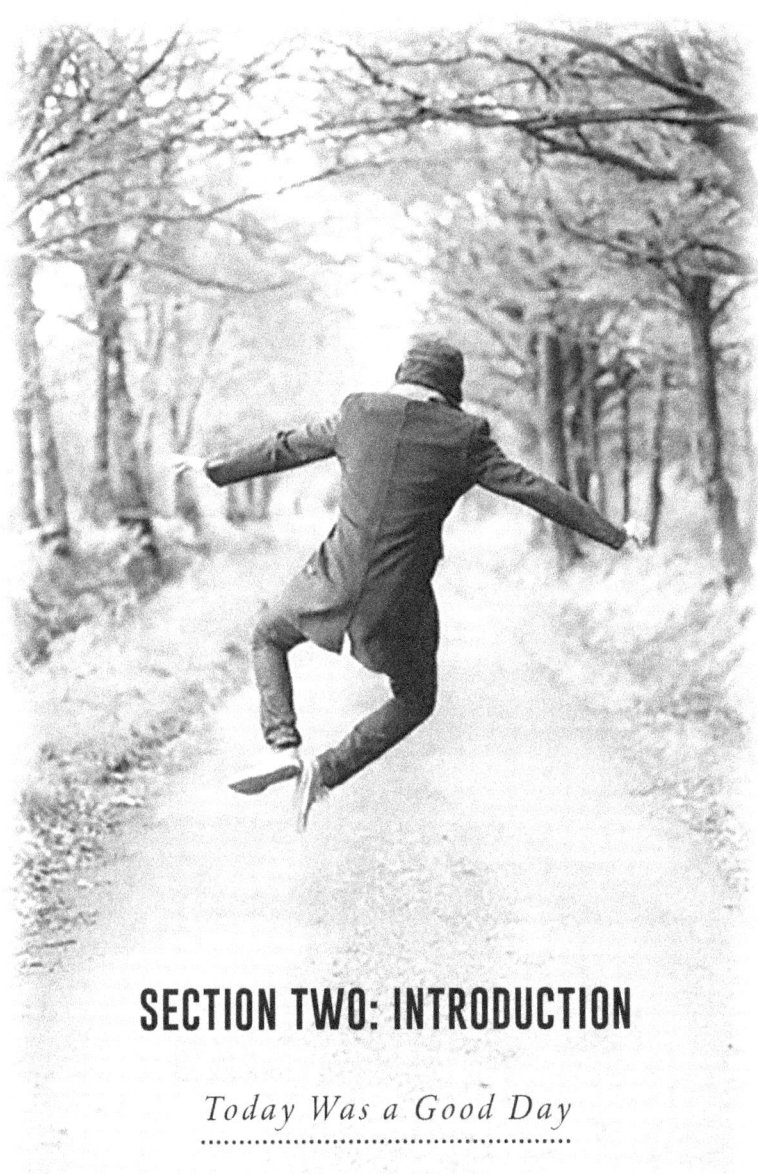

SECTION TWO: INTRODUCTION

Today Was a Good Day

Section 2 takes scenarios and lessons from the doctor-patient interaction arena. This section, entitled "Today Was a Good Day," seeks to provide a means to find worth and fulfillment in the things that all of us do daily. Of course, at the end of the day, we want to look back on the day and say these very words.

Section Two

This section examines the interactions between physicians and patients as a means to focus on specific communication and lifestyle issues that pertain to all people. This section has the same title as the first essay in the section, as well as the title of the book. This is for good reason. We want good days. We all want to feel good about ourselves. We want to be fulfilled. This section strives to utilize selected scenarios to highlight ways that all of us can end our day with the feeling that it, indeed, 'was a good day.'

Let us begin with an interaction between a patient with cancer and a physician.

Section Two

Essay 1
Today Was a Good Day

"Don't worry, it will get better" is a not uncommon prototypical physician utterance during a conversation between a physician and patient. Oftentimes, such is true, but when dealing with a seriously ill patient, such as a cancer patient, more often than not such is not true. Why, then, do we humans utter these words of unfounded encouragement and veiled optimism, when we know they are not true?

Most humans feel uncomfortable confronting a tearful emotional person, particularly when the expression of emotion is connected to a circumstance of such an immense magnitude as terminal cancer (a cancer that will eventually lead to the death of the patient). In the moment, what could be more assuring and comforting than the words "Don't worry, it will get better. We will overcome!" In the short term, these words comfort both the patient and the physician. In the long term, though, only the physician is comforted. The physician may see the patient one time only. If such is the case, the physician can walk out of the room after the conversation unscathed. If there exists a long-term relationship between the patient and the physician, those words may eventually adversely affect their relationship. "Doctor, you told me it would get better!"

Although the patient, perhaps with metastatic breast cancer, may feel comforted after the initial conversation, the harsh reality associated with the terminal nature of the disease eventually "catches up" to her. At that point, the patient and family begin passing through the five stages of grief, as outlined by Elisabeth Kubler-Ross (author of the seminal book *On Death and Dying*). There are several problems associated with the statement "Don't worry, it will get better." First and foremost, such a statement, when not true, sets the stage for further conveyances of "innocent non-truths" that can lead to, and often foster, suboptimal decision making. The patient and family can only make reasonable and rational decisions when they are dealing with the truth— with the facts. Decisions regarding surgical, medical or radiation therapy management,

Section Two

as well as decisions regarding end-of-life care, rely on accurate information such as the fact that the disease is terminal, a reasonable estimate of life expectancy, and the risks associated with the variety of available treatment options. A liberal transmission of accurate information regarding the diagnosis, best guess regarding predicted responses to treatments and prognosis (projected outcome) are key here. Realism and not pessimism or optimism should be the "fundamental rule of conversation etiquette" as it unfolds; and such should be the foundation of all subsequent conversations, as well. The withholding of such information due to suboptimal physician comfort level can, and often does, lead to the making of bad decisions. To be clear, one of the most common transgressions in this domain relates to what is not said. The uncomfortable nature of discussing the patient's mortality ("You will eventually succumb to this tumor") makes this portion of the discussion difficult to broach. However, to discuss is to educate. This leads to better decisions regarding end-of-life decisions. For both the patient and physician, it is not good to be either an optimist or pessimist here. It is always best to be a realist.

Another problem associated with "sugarcoating" the implications of the diagnosis or condition up front is related to the fact that when the truth really hits, it hits hard and can complicate subsequent emotional management. Emotional distress is best prevented and managed via confronting the truth.

Finally, uttering non-truths can undermine trust and the bond between the physician and the patient and family. Such a bond is secured by the employment of empathic conversations that are based on honesty. A comfort level that is founded on mutual trust is vital.

Let us dig deeper into the real reason the physician states "Don't worry, it will get better." The physician, like all humans, seeks comfort. The delivering of bad news is very uncomfortable for most people, including physicians. In addition, sitting with a tearful patient is uncomfortable for most mortals. As such, the physician, when confronted with such a situation, often seeks to end the uncomfortableness by patting the patient on the shoulder and uttering words of support that imply that *it will be alright*, when in reality it won't. This situation represents a lost opportunity to educate and comfort in a different way. By the latter, I mean by using tried-and-true com-

Section Two

munication skills, the most important of which is listening. Remember, an emotional patient may often not speak for an extended period of time. The physician may have trouble dealing with the silence that is only broken by sobs. He/she may then speak, with or without false assurances. The breaking of the silence, without question, alters the trajectory of the conversation. It most often diverts the conversation to something much less meaningful and less cathartic to the patient than the confrontation of facts and the truth. Physicians should wait for the patient to speak. The patient will, in less time than one might think, speak. What the patient utters will most certainly be revealing and meaningful.

Of course, the outlining of the entire spectrum of prognoses and treatment strategies is likely not appropriate at the first visit, unless confronted with an emergency situation. A rational and honest "shot across the bow" can set the stage for future conversations that ultimately lead to sound decision making based on the facts, not on untruths and misconceptions.

The conveyance of facts (the truth), while providing comfort (empathy) and ensuring that the physician will be there as a team member to help get through the ordeal, is invaluable ("We will get through this together"). As taught by Rabbi Kushner (author of *When Bad Things Happen to Good People*), dying patients are fearful of two things: pain and abandonment. Like it or not, patients put physicians on pedestals. Hence, the physician's honest guidance through the abyss associated with the making of tough informed decisions and often complex, painful and complication-ridden treatments is both needed and appreciated. Accompanying the patient through this most difficult journey is a far cry from abandonment (more on this later in Section 2, Essay 9).

So, the gentle empathic conveyance of the notion that "It may not get better" provides an honest and thoughtful introduction to what may be a long relationship between patient and physician, as well as with many non-medical interactions between two people. This is not to say that terminal patients should not strive and even fight for meaningfulness and fulfillment in what remains of their lives. They should, and their physicians should help them.

Helping the cancer patient and his/her family through difficult times, or for that matter anyone helping another through difficult times, can be extremely rewarding.

Section Two

Such interactions, and the gratitude that often emanates from them, should cause all of us to act accordingly and then say to oneself, as the day comes to an end, "Today was a good day!"

Section Two

....

Essay 2
....
*Is Your Life's Work a Calling?
Lessons from Global Neurosurgery*

In my relatively extensive international travels, I remain in perpetual awe regarding the quality of neurosurgery practiced worldwide. As I meander through the abyss of the worldwide neurosurgery community, I am constantly reminded of the impressive dedication to excellence by neurosurgeons in all reaches of the world. By and large, neurosurgeons worldwide practice their craft, often without adequate resources and under suboptimal conditions. More often than not, they practice their craft selflessly, with relative disregard for individual economic and "academic" rewards. What is it that makes neurosurgeons tick? What are the factors that stimulate them to, in many cases, overcome substantial barriers and obstacles, without significant regard for self (selflessness)?

I address in the essay that follows in this section (Section 2, Essay 3), the balancing of selflessness and selfishness. Here, I address the selflessness component in isolation. Regardless of the need to achieve some sort of a balance here (i.e., a work/life balance), the "giving" side of most (but not all) neurosurgeons is impressive and commendable. Again, why?

Is it the complexity of what neurosurgeons do? Does the devastating nature of many of the diseases and pathologies neurosurgeons treat draw them emotionally to an inner mission/giving core ethos? Or do they simply complete their tasks that are presented to them on a daily basis? Perhaps the true answer lies within the compelling book by Paul Kalanithi *When Breath Becomes Air,* which I referenced and discussed in Section 1, Essay 4. In view of its compelling nature, I am referencing it again. This book has many life lessons for neurosurgeons and non-neurosurgeons alike. Kalanithi was a neurosurgery resident (neurosurgery trainee) who died of cancer just prior to his graduation from neurosurgery residency. In the book, he relates the following story related to the changing of a mission-like statement for medical students at Stanford University. "…several students argued for the removal of the language insisting we

Section Two

place our patients' interests above our own. The rest of us didn't allow this discussion to continue for long. The words stayed. This kind of egotism struck me as antithetical to medicine and, it should be noted, entirely reasonable. Indeed, this is how 99 percent of people select their jobs: pay, work environment, hours. But that's the point. Putting lifestyle first is how you find a job—not a calling." Hence, I came to the conclusion that neurosurgeons who "give" to their patients and work more than they receive, approach their craft not as a job but rather as a calling.

For those neurosurgeons so inclined, be proud of yourselves. All non-neurosurgeons so inclined, likewise, be proud of yourselves. We can all learn from those who give so much and receive so little in return. The global neurosurgery community is but one of many, many examples of people treating their job or life's work as a calling. In a way, this is how true leaders are made

Section Two

Essay 3
Selflessness and Selfishness

In this essay, I focus on neurosurgeons. Nevertheless, there are lessons for all to be had. Many neurosurgeons are, in a way, martyrs. They give of themselves to their patients. They sacrifice free time and time with family for their patients. They, and other critical care oriented medical professionals, are frequently awakened from a deep sleep to hear of a patient crisis and all too frequently are beckoned to roll out of bed to attend to the needs of a patient. Very few other professions, be they medical or nonmedical, expect so much from their practitioners (my biased opinion).

I emphasize that such giving of oneself to others is expected in the neurosurgical world. It is an unspoken dictum in the neurosurgery community—i.e., neurosurgery organizations, neurosurgery mentors and peers. It is also expected by patients. Finally and most importantly, it is expected by neurosurgeons themselves. Neurosurgeons can be their own strictest of taskmasters, though. Oftentimes, they take their sacrifices to an extreme—an extreme that smacks of machismo. The macho neurosurgeon does more surgical cases, takes on more duties, works more hours, and spends more time away from home than is, perhaps, necessary. In some cases, a focus on **how much** a neurosurgeon does (i.e., number of surgical cases) overtakes a focus on **how much good** the neurosurgeon does.

Regardless of the rationale for the sacrifices neurosurgeons' make, such selfless behavior takes its toll. Fractured relationships, divorce, missing a substantial portion of their children's growth and development, and burnout can wear on the neurosurgeon to the extent that the protective shell of mental toughness that is characteristic of neurosurgeons is challenged, often threatened and occasionally shattered.

Although, to a degree, neurosurgeons are appropriately expected to be selfless, they must also take on a healthy amount of some sort of counter-measure to compensate for their *selfless* behavior. For the purposes of discussion here, I call this counter-measure *selfishness*. Selfishness is generally considered to be a negative attribute—a

Section Two

behavior that is to be avoided. It is also deemed as socially inappropriate in most circumstances. But, if selfishness is modified and internalized, it can be a very useful tool; i.e., a counter-measure to temper selflessness. Such a *selflessness/selfishness* balance or see-saw can be thought of as another way of looking at *work/life balance*. Every neurosurgeon knows and should admit that, with a little more effort and focus, they could go home earlier most evenings. They also know that there are times when a partner can take on a case or two if said partner is less busy. Unfortunately, it also becomes all too easy to *hang out* at the hospital, rather than going home. The hospital, in reality, is a very comfortable place for neurosurgeons. Analogous situations in other professions obviously exist and must be managed accordingly.

There are many, many more examples of excessive selfless behaviors. They are everywhere and they permeate all aspects of the life of neurosurgeons and non-neurosurgeons alike. Selfishly rectifying and neutralizing these acts of excessive selflessness can help all of us adjust and react to the stresses that life throws our way. It can reduce burnout, help restore and help heal fractured relationships and allow us to watch our kids and our grandchildren grow up.

I ask the following question of all neurosurgeons, and all other humans. Have you ever gone home early, if such is possible in your line of work, and felt guilty—hoping that one of your partners or coworkers did not see you slip out the door? If so, get a little more selfish and go home early more often—that is, if your job allows and you have completed your work. Equally importantly, encourage your partners and coworkers to do the same. We all must realize that it is not a crime to go home when the work is done. Finally, we should diminish our focus on, and perhaps obsession, with **how much** we do (i.e., number of surgical cases or the volume of product produced) and reorient our focus to **how much good** we do and the **quality of our product**. Hopefully, then, we can all go home earlier **and** simultaneously feel better about ourselves.

Section Two

Essay 4
Mismatched Expectations

When two individuals interact with the purpose of crafting "a plan," assumptions and preconceived notions inevitably lead to expectations regarding "the plan." Most often, expectations are aligned. However, if one expects an outcome that is not aligned with the expectation of the other participant, one or both may be disappointed with the end result.

This not uncommonly occurs during the operative decision-making process and the attainment of the operative consent for a neurosurgical procedure. For example, a patient with myelopathy (weakness and balance problems emanating from spinal cord compression) and neck pain may benefit from spinal cord decompression (relief of compression) and, possibly, a fusion (spine stabilization, most often with screws and rods or plates)—depending on the circumstances.

The surgeon "sees" a patient with significant signs of spinal cord compression (pressure on the spinal cord). The patient may have fallen several times; hence, he/she is at risk for further spinal cord injury as a result of such. The patient "feels" neck pain and complains predominantly of neck pain. He/she is not so concerned about the myelopathy (weakness and balance issues).

Obviously, the expectations of the surgeon and the patient are not aligned. Postoperatively, the patient's myelopathy (spinal cord dysfunction) improves, but the neck pain may not. If such is the case, the patient's "Health-Related Quality of Life" (HRQOL) metrics (an assessment of the effect of treatment on physical function and pain) may not improve. The surgeon is elated with the clinical result (improved myelopathy; i.e., balance and fine motor skill improvement), but the patient continues to complain of neck pain and fails to "see" the clinical improvement that elates the surgeon.

This is a common scenario for surgeons and their patients, particularly spine surgeons. So, how does one manage expectations so that the aforementioned scenario can be avoided? I suggest a three-part strategy:

Section Two

1. Each participant should know the expectations of the other participant.
2. The participants should alter the expectations so that they are aligned. This often involves compromise.
3. Accordingly, craft and execute a plan.

Know the Expectations

Simply discuss the expectations preoperatively. "Your surgery is designed to deal with your balance and fine motor skill issues but may not relieve your neck pain."

Alter the Expectations so that They Are Aligned

If expectations cannot be aligned, an alternative strategy may be in order. "If you understand that neck pain may not be resolved with surgery, are you okay with proceeding to address the balance issues and fine motor skills deficits?"

Accordingly, Craft a Plan

If the surgeon and patient cannot come to an agreement regarding surgery-related expectations, a tough decision may be in order. If persistent or worsened postoperative pain is unacceptable, perhaps the planned surgery is not for this patient—at least at this time. The patient can choose to avoid or delay surgery. While this is not optimal, it provides a choice for the patient. It, indeed, is preferable to having to choose from two suboptimal options. Such is better than being surprised by an unanticipated outcome. As an aside, patients who are given treatment options from which to choose, become empowered to help direct their own care. This is a powerful and integral component of the clinical decision-making process—i.e., shared decision making.

By optimizing expectation management, neurosurgeons can improve patient satisfaction and, equally importantly, surgeon satisfaction. After all, a happy patient makes for a happy doctor. Isn't this how all "give and take" interactions should work, for all of us? This is a lesson that can employed universally. With a mutually aligned set of expectations that are associated with an interaction between two individuals, both parties should be happy with the result. Advice to all: Align expectations!

Section Two

Essay 5
Curiosity and Listening

The gift of curiosity and the art of listening are two of the most important tools in the armamentarium of anyone who desires to communicate effectively. Without question, such should resonate with all of us. We all perpetually communicate. Such is an obligatory component of investigative diagnostic "detective work" for the neurosurgeon, but the importance of curiosity as a learning tool transcends all professions and lifestyles. The gift of curiosity can be developed and nurtured as each of us finds our way through our individual lives. As curiosity increases, the "drive" to answer questions intensifies and the pursuit of answers, diagnoses, and solutions becomes what one may consider a "healthy obsession." To be appropriately curious is a virtue.

The strategies we employ to go about harnessing our curiosity is critical, though. With curiosity, the neurosurgeon examines the patient, sorts through images and other diagnostic tests, and often discusses the aforementioned with colleagues. This is no different than the strategy used by all humans to solve problems; i.e., to develop management strategies, and communicate with colleagues. Hence, we should listen and listen carefully. Physicians take a history. They listen to the patient's story. They seek family members' version of the story. They listen to nurses, medical assistants, and many others.

The question, however, is—do we really listen? Do we listen enough? Does the neurosurgeon let the patient tell the entire story? Do the rest of us truly "hear" what others want us to know? Do we allow others to express their concerns, their thoughts, and their fears?

We humans naturally want to fix things. We often think we know what's best for ourselves and for others. But do we? Unless we truly listen to each other and allow our counterpart to tell the complete story, we may miss important diagnostic (in the case of the neurosurgeon) or emotional cues. Silence on our part, which is a key to good listening, can cause the patient (in the case of a conversation with a neurosurgeon) to express critical emotions (e.g., tearfulness), unearth hidden concerns,

Section Two

or uncover key diagnostic cues. This translates to all interactions. Our instinctual desire to "fix things" can, however, interfere with the deployment of listening as our most important problem-solving tools. We often interrupt, thus changing the trajectory of the conversation. We, perhaps, interrupt because we are uncomfortable. The counterpart in the conversation may have been on the verge of providing incredibly important information that may now remain forever hidden.

In the spine surgery domain, my subspecialty, we are often embarrassingly inaccurate regarding patient selection for surgery. Why is this, you might ask? Perhaps because we base our strategic clinical plan on the foundation of a "wrong diagnosis." If we ask the right questions, and then truly listen, we may come to understand that the patient's real problem is not related to the imaging finding but in reality is associated with a non-surgical diagnosis.

Some time back, my wife and I were walking along a street and passed a café that had a sign out front that read something like this (I refer to this scenario in other chapters in this book as well):

"Coffee: $5.
Coffee, with a hello: $2.
Coffee, with a hello, how are you?: $1."

How wonderful! We so often forget to engage people with simple yet meaningful conversation. The most important part of this message, though, is unspoken. Once we ask the question "How are you?"—we must listen! We must focus on the answer to the question—i.e., how they are. We learn so much by listening and so little by talking.

We must all seek to master the art of listening. Our colleagues, our family, and our coworkers will provide valuable information if we simply let them. Soooooo, we should strive to be curious, ask open-ended questions, and then listen. Only then can we see the all-too-often-present "elephant in the room; ie, the finding or emotion that can only be uncovered by listening."

Section Two

Essay 6
Boundaries

Boundaries are everywhere. They permeate all layers of communication, politics, and social and personal belief arenas. Boundaries between nations or properties may be of little meaning to the friendly neighbors on either side of the boundary, or they may represent reason for strife if violated in situations where hostility and disdain divide the juxtaposed neighbors.

We all have individual boundaries as well. Some are "enforced" more than others. Boundaries, at one extreme, may be blurry and are often minimally enforced or are ignored, or they may be distinct and clear cut at the other extreme—and, as such, are often strictly enforced. Bottom line, boundaries may be of trivial or of critical significance.

The consideration of boundaries, as they pertain to a neurosurgeon's interactions with patients, may be of greater significance than most realize. In the outpatient or inpatient milieu, in which crucial conversations are often held between a patient and a physician, boundary considerations can be divided into two distinct domains: 1) boundary establishment and 2) boundary management.

With most conversations between a patient and a neurosurgeon, "soft" unspoken boundaries are assumed. These include a myriad of self-imposed boundaries that essentially pertain to common decency and respect for others. The expectations of participants in the vast majority of conversations are that each participant will exhibit an acceptable sense of decorum during the conversation. When, for example, an insult is conveyed by one of the two conversation participants, a boundary has been crossed—and, hence, must now be managed.

A physician should NEVER insult a patient (such should be extended to us all—physicians and non-physicians alike), but if a patient insults a physician, the physician must enter into a boundary management mode. Again, such is true for us all. He/she should rise above it all by remaining calm, let the patient or conversation participant vent, and then—after the venting is finished—calmly address the concerns that lead

Section Two

to the "conversation derailment." Further argument and disagreement/discord will only fuel the fire.

There are many, many types and examples of boundary establishment and management. I am going to focus on an example relating to drug-seeking behavior. If a physician believes, as do I, that the long-term use of narcotic medication in a chronic pain syndrome patient escalates the magnitude of the pain syndrome, boundary setting may be in order. If boundaries are not set early in the conversation, soft boundaries may be crossed due to the lack of clarity regarding boundaries. The patient may have very different expectations from the visit than does the physician; i.e., opiate prescription versus denial of such. Strife may arise in such a scenario. In such cases, lack of clarity fosters potential conflict. This applies to all conversations in which soft boundaries and mismatched expectations exist.

The scenario was initiated and fostered by insufficient or suboptimal boundary establishment. The patient may not be in a position, or is not willing, to set boundaries here, but the physician is. If the physician makes it clear to the patient up front that he/she does not prescribe narcotics, the patient's expectations will undoubtedly be modified. Such can be accomplished with the citing or provision of literature supporting the physician's position, signage in the outpatient clinic, or by simple verbal communication of the physician's philosophy at the outset of the conversation.

The establishment of a boundary, however, does not ensure that boundary-related strife will not occur. This is where boundary management enters the fray. The establishment of a clear-cut boundary, such as a "no narcotic prescription rule," does not guarantee that the patient will willingly accept his/her rejection of a narcotic prescription request. Regardless, in this situation, the boundary that was set can now be managed.

Management options for this boundary conflict include patient education and discussion regarding chronic pain and how it is best managed. Such a discussion should involve the long term risks of long term narcotic use, including escalation, not de-escalation of the intensity of the pain. Regardless, such a discussion can be difficult and may often end in a dead lock, with the two sides unable or unwilling to meet in the middle.

Section Two

Of note, the "middle" here, as it is with many conflict conversations, is an interesting place. To the physician, the patient should seek more appropriate means of managing pain. To the patient, the physician should simply prescribe narcotics to manage the pain. Hence, boundary management strategy development may need to be taken to the next level—i.e., ethical considerations. By this, I very simply mean that the physician might consider conveying to the patient that he/she is committed to "doing what's right." All physicians have either taken an oath or abide by such—i.e., the Hippocratic oath that applies the essence of the Latin phrase "Primum non nocere" (First do no harm). In the spirit of clarity, the Hippocratic oath includes the phrase "to abstain from doing harm" (**Greek**: ἐπὶ δηλήσει δὲ καὶ ἀδικίῃ εἴρξειν). If I, as a physician, believe that narcotic medication will harm the patient, I cannot in good conscience prescribe such for the patient. Hence, the physician "abstained from doing harm."

Although the patient may remain dissatisfied with the conversation, the discussion is over. In this case, a boundary was set and managed. The physician did what he/she believes is the ethical and right thing to do, and hopefully the patient will be guided to a better place regarding his/her care by such actions.

On a much more common and real-life scenario is experienced by those of us who have raised or are raising children. Parents know that the setting of expectations and boundaries up front is much more effective than attempting to set expectations and boundaries after an infraction has occurred.

We all need to establish and manage boundaries in all aspects of our lives. This process must be driven by a legitimate concern for the wellbeing of the other conversant and, of course, our own wellbeing. We all must remember—"First do no harm." By setting boundaries, we are more likely 'to do what's right. These examples provide lessons for us all in our quest to avoid unnecessary strife.

Section Two

Essay 7
On Being Judgmental

"Do not judge, or you too will be judged. For in the same way you judge others, you will be judged, and with the measure you use, it will be measured to you."
— Matthew 7:1-2

We all routinely judge others and their actions. Such is inevitable. Judging is a "product" of assessment. We usually keep such assessments and judgments to ourselves, though. We judge, but are not judgmental. We do not convey our judgments and assessments to others—and, most specifically, to those who we are judging. In the course of everyday conversation, the act of expressing judgment (and thus becoming judgmental) is in a sense an expression of self-superiority. "I am better than you." "I am right, and you are wrong." "I have taken the high road and you the low road."

Regarding our interactions with our family, friends, and colleagues, the expression of judgment can have unintended consequences. These include a deterioration of trust, a degradation of the relationship and an alteration of the "trajectory" of the conversation. I would like to focus here on the latter, as it relates to physician-patient interactions and relationships.

Let's create a hypothetical scenario here, in which a physician is acquiring a history from a patient. In the course of the conversation, the patient states that he drinks at least a liter of vodka every day. This may be shocking to the physician, but the physician's response becomes a pivotal point in this patient-physician interaction. The physician could A) not respond and continue the collection of patient-related information or B) respond by conveying a gesture of disapproval or a statement admonishing such behavior. With A), the neurosurgeon is not judgmental, but with B), the surgeon is conveying judgment, and hence is judgmental.

Section Two

Such judgment expression can be detrimental to both the conversation between the physician and patient and the outcome of the conversation. The expression of judgment immediately conveys a sense of disapproval to the patient. This, in turn, may, and often does, change the "trajectory" of the conversation—from one of information gathering from a willing source (the patient), to a conversation in which the source (the patient) is less willing to accurately inform the physician.

The conveyance of judgment (the act of being judgmental) does two things. First, it in a sense is an expression of self-superiority ("I am better than you." "I am right and you are wrong." "I have taken the high road and you the low road."). This is a very slippery slope and represents a "place" that none of us should go. Second, it diminishes the meaningfulness of the subsequent conversation and the gathering of data by the physician. The patient will be less likely to be honestly forthcoming in response to future questions.

Physicians must remain "judgment neutral" during interactions with patients. They must gather accurate information and use such for the betterment of the patient's overall quality of life and outcome. Knowing that a patient drinks a liter of vodka each day is useful information. Physicians should accept such information at its face value and then act accordingly to lead the patient to a better place in a "calculated manner." Bottom line, we cannot help judging, but we can refrain from being judgmental.

All of us, physicians and non-physicians alike, in the course of daily activities, come across similar or parallel situations and scenarios. Whether the conversation participants are physician-patient, friend-friend, colleague-colleague, or parent-child, the passing of judgment, i.e. the act of being judgmental, can inadvertently alter the trajectory of the conversation and lead to unwanted and untoward outcomes.

Section Two

Essay 8
To Teach Is to Give

"Education is the most powerful weapon we can use to change the world."
– Nelson Mandela

Teaching is an art form—an art form in which the teacher gives to the learner. This art form is operationalized (brought to life) in a variety of ways, ranging from the teaching of children at home and in the classroom to the much more subtle "teaching by example." In a way, medical journals, such as the journal I edit, **WORLD NEUROSURGERY,** should be thought of as a platform for teaching. In this essay, I focus on **WORLD NEUROSURGERY** as an example. There are many more examples outside of medicine. Regardless, authors of submitted manuscripts teach the consumer/readers. Readers then teach each other and are perhaps inspired to write (and teach) themselves. The process becomes cyclical, as more and more surgeons are attracted to the cycle of teaching and learning. Hence, there will be a never-ending source of new ideas and concepts; if you will, an infinite reservoir of innovation that leads to thinking, action and teaching more innovation.

The publication of scientific manuscripts is a very complicated and complex process. Nelson Mandela's quote *"Education is the most powerful weapon we can use to change the world"* appropriately puts the mission of **WORLD NEUROSURGERY** into perspective. We hope to enlighten through education so that neurosurgeons from all corners of the world learn from the myriad of messages passed on through the multiple avenues provided by **WORLD NEUROSURGERY**.

Of note, however, is that this is not a simple process. What goes into a published or, for that matter, a rejected, manuscript is an entire additional level of teaching and learning. The reviewers and the section editors bear a huge responsibility to not only make determinations regarding the viability of a manuscript, but also bear a huge responsibility to teach the authors. This is irrespective of the ultimate status of the manuscript—i.e., rejection vs. acceptance. The authors deserve and should expect a thoughtful critique that, in a very real sense, is a learning experience for the author and teaching experience for the reviewer and section editor.

There, however, is indeed another layer of complexity. Reviewers and section editors learn by reviewing manuscripts and, ultimately, learn from teaching via their critical appraisal of manuscripts. I guess that this is not so unusual. After all, teaching is one of the highest forms of learning, and as eloquently stated by Matthea Harvey, *"Teaching is a great way to keep learning."* Being a good teacher implies that the teacher harbors an acquired mastery of the subject matter. In a very real sense, the act of teaching causes the teacher to learn and increase the level of the acquired mastery of the subject matter.

A quote from Socrates helps us put all of this into perspective: *"I cannot teach anybody anything. I can only make them think."* Put another way, *"I cannot teach you anything, the most I can hope to achieve is to cause you to learn."* "Causing to learn" is a key operative here. The act of "causing to learn" must obligatorily take place in an "enriched environment."

Teaching and learning are optimized when practiced in an "enriched environment." I would like to think that **WORLD NEUROSURGERY** fosters the development and perpetuation of such an enriched environment. We are all learners and teachers. Oftentimes, we are simultaneously both. By employing the complicated web of learning and teaching portrayed above in a friendly and structured environment that fosters information transmission, **WORLD NEUROSURGERY** has created a platform for learning and teaching that is indeed enriched.

In summary, I have several messages:

> **To the authors of neurosurgical publications and all other publications as well**: Keep it coming. Keep writing. Take criticism as a constructive teaching aid. It is meant to be a means for you to learn.

> **To the reviewers and section editors:** Continue to provide meaningful feedback and constructive criticism for each manuscript, no

Section Two

matter how good or how bad it may be. The authors deserve such and can learn from your priceless words of wisdom.

To all neurosurgeons: Let us each do our part to foster and nurture our enriched environment at ***WORLD NEUROSURGERY***. With the entire team harboring the same goals, ***WORLD NEUROSURGERY*** will continue to grow into its place/position as a dominant reservoir of education for all neurosurgeons worldwide.

To all of us, neurosurgeons and non-neurosurgeons alike, there exists innumerable opportunities to teach and to learn. Such occurs, almost always, in an enriched environment. We all should seek to teach and to absorb when taught. To teach is to give, and to learn is to open the door to the knowledge that flows from teaching. The onus on all of us is to keep this vibrant interaction between teaching and learning alive and thriving.

Section Two

Essay 9
Doctor, Do Not Abandon Your Patient

"Dying patients are afraid of two things: pain and abandonment."
– Rabbi Kushner

Roughly thirty years ago, I was caring for a patient with metastatic breast cancer to the spine (breast cancer with daughter tumors that have invaded the spine). She was young, in her early thirties. She was a kind and gentle person, but for some reason she enjoyed few visits from family and friends. I performed a complex decompression and spinal reconstruction procedure for her and, shortly thereafter, left for the American Association of Neurological Surgeons meeting. It was at this meeting that I heard a wonderful and inspiring talk by Rabbi Harold S. Kushner, author of the book *When Bad Things Happen to Good People*. His talk was complex, yet beautifully articulated. He spoke of death, dying, living, disappointment, tragedy and much more. He also spoke specifically to the audience of neurosurgeons—commenting on the fact that people/patients put neurosurgeons on pedestals, whether they like it or not. He also uttered these words: "Dying patients are afraid of two things: pain and abandonment." Considering my recent encounter with my metastatic breast cancer patient, Rabbi Kushner's talk hit me like a ton of bricks. When I returned from the meeting and visited my patient, she had remained alone and without visitors by reports from the nursing staff. We talked. I asked if I could sit at her side. She said, "Of course." We then began an ongoing dialogue about our lives and what made each of us tick. We talked about her future and her pain. Yes, I treated her pain, but more importantly we talked. These visits happened twice daily until her discharge. The time spent was trivial in the big scheme of things. What was of utmost importance, though, was the fact that she could count on my twice-daily visits and our dialogue. She didn't need a lot of my time, simply the assurance that I cared about her as a human being, and that I was not abandoning her.

Section Two

This entire ordeal was a life-changing experience for me. I can only hope that our interactions were meaningful to her as well. I think they were…. No, I know they were.

What did I take home from this experience? I came to the realization that I must always make time to talk to my patients, particularly those who are at high risk of fearing abandonment. We might talk about anything: their disease, their expectations, their family, my family. This also was one of my first life lessons regarding the art of listening. Sometimes it is best to let others talk, letting them take the conversation to places previously unknown, but nearly always revealing and enlightening. With such interactions, neurosurgeons have the opportunity to let their patients know that they are human. More importantly, however, we can and should make it perfectly clear that we will work together with the patient and family as a team to fight the disease at hand. The patient, hence, should then feel secure, without a concern regarding physician abandonment.

So, thank you, Rabbi Kushner. You taught us all a very important life lesson: *Don't abandon our patients!* For non-physicians, don't abandon each other. Rabbi Kushner, for the lessons you taught us, we are eternally grateful.

Section Two

Essay 10
Suffering

Suffering takes on many forms; ranging from the end-result of "man's inhumanity to man" to an emotional response associated with disability or pain. The former is, unfortunately, a commonplace occurrence in our world today. So many suffer at the hands of tyrants, whose genocidal actions inflict misery that is associated with significant suffering and loss. For lack of better terms, let's call the former "third-world suffering" and the latter "first-world suffering." In many respects regarding those who suffer in the first-world sense, suffering comes as a choice. Such first-world sufferers are often demonstrative regarding their disability or pain, thus in a way sharing/inflicting/imposing the emotions associated with their pain or disability on and to others. Alternatively, they could hide or shield their "pain" from others, while focusing on managing the pain. Clinical pain psychologists use this strategy as a tool to help patients with chronic pain syndromes. In such patients, their pain becomes an interface between the patient and the rest of the world, including friends, family, and healthcare providers. Their pain interferes with communication, friendships, relationships, and life in general. The goal of the clinical pain psychologist, in large part, is to cause the patient to shift the experience of pain, and its associated emotions, from the position of an intrusive interface with others (in front of the patient's face) to a position off to the side—where the patient can begin to manage, study and learn about the pain and what makes it worse and what makes it better, while at the same time permitting the patient to interact with the others as if there were no suffering. The choice to shield the awareness of the pain from others and to learn from the pain facilitates and nurtures a healing process by overcoming self-pity. "Laugh and the world laughs with you. Cry and you cry alone."

When a neurosurgeon identifies a "first-world chronic pain patient," he/she should strive to get the patient to a better place. Neurosurgeons, however, do not have the time nor the skillset required to effectively intervene here. Seeking assistance from

Section Two

pain psychologists or other professionals in the cognitive behavioral therapy domain may be very helpful. If such a professional is not available, a show of empathy and understanding can go a long way. Encouraging increased, rather than decreased, activity (do more, not less) and discussing the fact that although activity may induce pain, the pain is not an indicator or harbinger of harm (explaining the differentiation between hurt and harm) is a start. With such a show of compassion and empathy, the surgeon can at least attempt to initiate the road to recovery. We must remember, "first-world" sufferers are truly miserable people. The least he/she can do is lend a helpful hand, however small that that hand may be.

Section Two

Essay 11
Facing Rejection

All of us have faced rejection. In fact, some neurosurgeons may have received a letter from me that informed them of a manuscript rejection by **World Neurosurgery** (I am Editor-in-Chief of **World Neurosurgery**). Such may have read as follows:

> Dear Vik,
> I am very disappointed that we are unable to accept your paper for publication. Via consensus, the reviewers recommend rejection.
>
> The Editorial Board is hopeful that you will find their comments constructive and edifying. Please consider the reviews as a suggestion to modify or rewrite your manuscript and resubmit elsewhere. We sincerely hope that this process has been of academic benefit for you.
>
> We appreciate your support of **WORLD NEUROSURGERY** and look forward to further submissions from you in the future.
>
> Regretfully,
> Edward C. Benzel, M.D.
> Editor-in-Chief

This letter was sent to Vikram Prabhu, a reviewer and section editor for **World Neurosurgery**. His paper was rejected; however, his response to rejection was quite unique and, in fact, extraordinarily admirable:

> Dear Ed:
> Thanks for taking a look at the manuscript for us and considering it. The reviewers' comments are both insightful and very helpful. I do appreciate it….

Section Two

> *I feel it reflects the high quality and ethical review process of* **World Neurosurgery** *and I feel very privileged to be associated with it.*
>
> Vik

We can all look at glasses as being either half full or half empty. Vik looked at this glass as being half full. He "saw" the review process as fair and constructive. He responded in a collegial manner that demonstrated his appreciation of the review process. I applaud him for the fact that he responded, as well as for the nature of his response.

Rejection is never easy, but when faced with rejection the way in which we respond, in a very real way, is a measure of integrity and character. As the Editor-in-Chief of **World Neurosurgery**, I receive many responses from authors regarding rejection. Most involve inquiry or clarification. Some are reflective of rejection associated anger. Vik's response was unique and, I might say, most appreciated. It represents an example, and a template, for all of us as we respond to rejection and constructive negative feedback. Responding with character is the key/ ie, receiving the criticism as constructive—not destructive.

Thank you, Vikram Prabhu, for responding with character. You are a good man!

Section Two

Essay 12

Emotional Health in the Midst of the Covid-19 Pandemic

I am not an expert on emotions, nor do I harbor a unique insight into the mental and emotional health of caregivers during the trying times of COVID-19 pandemic. I did, however, virtually communicate regularly (daily) with our residents, fellows, and some faculty at the Cleveland Clinic in Cleveland, Ohio, USA. Residents and fellows are trainees, in this case, in neurosurgery. Please note the Cleveland Ohio and the Northeast Ohio region of the United States was relatively spared a major surge from the COVID-19 pandemic. So, in Cleveland, Ohio, USA, we dealt with a relatively flat, but relatively prolonged low-level pandemic. In our environment, which was much less stressed than New York City, Northern Italy and other pockets of devastation around the world, we focused on caring for pandemic patients while placing the routine neurosurgery patient on the "back burner." Neurosurgeons played a limited role in the direct care of COVID-19 patients during the pandemic. Hence, they had time and technology to function in a virtual communication environment. They found the virtual platform for communication to be effective regarding information exchange. We established a daily lecture series for our trainees, had tumor boards, morbidity and mortality conferences, journal clubs (including multi-institutional journal clubs), specialty conferences, etc.—all virtual. Our faculty provided a newfound, and much appreciated, time to share their knowledge and expertise with the trainees. The "normal" daily grind often did not permit/provide sufficient time for such activities. Residents, fellows and faculty alike enjoyed this new opportunity for information transmission and exchange, and for the opportunity to share and conquer our individual emotional challenges.

This virtual communication platform also provided an avenue for talking through our concerns. In listening to the residents and fellows, I heard, and felt, many emotions emanating from their mouths. Perhaps the most prominent emotion "surfacing" during

Section Two

the pandemic was that of anxiety. An article by Shanafelt, Ripp and Trockel, published in *JAMA Viewpoint,* eloquently outlines the issues at hand as they pertain to the COVID-19 pandemic, associated anxieties, and its effect on healthcare providers (*JAMA Viewpoint,* April 7, 2020. *Understanding and Addressing Sources of Anxiety Among Health Care Professionals During the COVID-19 Pandemic.* Tait Shanafelt, M.D.; Jonathan Ripp, M.D., MPH; Mickey Trockel, M.D., Ph.D.). They address eight sources of anxiety that the pandemic unleashed: (1) often inadequate access to appropriate personal protective equipment, (2) being exposed to COVID-19 at work and taking the infection home to their family, (3) not having rapid access to testing if they developed COVID-19 symptoms and the concomitant fear of propagating infection at work, (4) uncertainty that their organization will support/take care of their personal and family needs if they develop infection, (5) access to childcare during increased work hours and school closures, (6) support for other personal and family needs as work hours and demands increased (food, hydration, lodging, transportation), (7) being able to provide competent medical care if deployed to a new area (e.g., non-ICU nurses having to function as ICU nurses), and (8) lack of access to up-to-date information and communication.

The authors then distilled the eight sources of anxiety into five fundamental requests or asks of healthcare professionals from their institutions: hear me, protect me, prepare me, support me, and care for me. Shanafelt et al go on to describe how institutional leaders can, and should be, up front and visibly provide both support and leadership as they guide their respective institutions through the abyss to address each and every one of the five asks. Shanafelt et al go on to state that institutional leaders "must encourage team members to ask for help when they need it and emphasize that health care professionals and leaders must rely on each other." Leaders should ensure that no one feels they must make difficult decisions alone. Healthcare professionals should also feel empowered to defer less important and time-sensitive activities, such as routine elective neurosurgery procedures. They closed by discussing gratitude. Hence, a final ask (6th ask) of the healthcare provider is introduced: "honor me." "Recognize and give me my due credit for my sacrifices."

We must also recognize, however, that other emotions well up within the minds of caregivers. From conversations with the residents and fellows at the Cleveland Clinic,

Section Two

emotions and feelings other than anxiety are described—and appeared to take an emotional toll on even the most stoic. These emotions and feelings fed off, and often amplified each other—somehow, eventually circling back to anxiety amplification in some way. Other than anxiety, fear and guilt seemed to be the most prominent emotions/feelings that have surfaced under the shroud of the COVID-19 pandemic. A second-year neurosurgery resident at the Cleveland Clinic at the time commented on the fear associated with the management of patients, whether COVID-19 positive or not. The fear associated with the unknown and the fact that a "silent killer" may be lurking can have profound emotional effects. "How can I ask my patients to trust me, if I am not sure that I can trust them? Is it wrong to worry about myself and about my family at home? How long will this remain our reality?" asked the resident. Rarely have neurosurgeons been afraid of their patients. Perhaps in the days of brain biopsies for HIV patients or for suspected Creutzfeldt-Jakob disease patients (diseases that could be transmitted to the surgeon and other healthcare providers) we faced a fear for our safety, but not with every patient we see and touch. Hence, we have rarely been concerned for our own safety, as well as the safety of our patients. In the minds of over-stressed trainees and staff neurosurgeons, the patient had become a threat to the neurosurgeons and their families.

And, what about the fear of associated potential retribution from the institution if one would have voiced concern over insufficient safety measures, such as personal protective equipment? Such fears and concerns surfaced in the national media. A fourth year neurosurgery resident at the Cleveland Clinic at the time) shared the anxiety provoking nature related to these concerns. "As a resident, there is fear of potential retribution for speaking up regarding the shortage of personal protective equipment and personal safety while caring for COVID-19 positive patients. Trainees across the country are checking in with one another and we hear multiple stories of residents being asked to choose between continued employment and reasonable requests for personal safety amidst a nationwide pandemic. The fear of punishment and potential termination only adds to the air of anxiety we are all dealing with during this time." These fears may be founded or unfounded, likely on an institution specific basis, but the fear was real, regardless. Residents and fellows are particularly vulnerable here. Their staff, teachers and mentors must protect and advise them in such circumstances.

Section Two

The aforementioned fears often resulted in guilt—guilt emanating from fears that, in a way, pit us (neurosurgeons and trainees) against the patient or against the institution. This isn't how it's supposed to be. We are supposed to be on the same side of the battle, fighting a disease together. We, during the pandemic, perhaps did not view it that way. How unfortunate.

Another second year neurosurgery resident at the Cleveland Clinic at the time articulated another form of guilt during the pandemic—a guilt associated with not doing enough. "I have felt a sense of guilt permeating my daily routine since COVID-19 interrupted our neurosurgical training. I chose neurosurgery, a highly sub-specialized field, in hopes of merging a love for the arts with a devotion to the service of others. What a better way, than to provide service in the reparation, protection, and study of the organ system at the origin of every piece of art ever created? Now, however, in light of a viral respiratory illness devastating non-neurosurgical populations, my choice of sub-specialties has resulted in flagrant discrepancy between my burgeoning neurosurgical duties/skillset and my desire to serve. The guilt that I felt is a mixture of sadness for the lives lost, frustration in feeling unable to assist, and shame at my inactivity while others are thrown into the fray. How can I mitigate the dissonance in this scenario? As of yet, I haven't established a perfect solution. For the time being, I am recommitting to daily neurosurgical study, to rediscovering my love for running and literature, and to the knowledge that the training I chose, while sub-specialized, will someday help me to serve future patients when, eventually, I am called to act."

This guilt was shared by one of her chief residents (a seventh-year resident at the Cleveland Clinic during the pandemic—the training program for Neurosurgery is seven years). She was emotionally connected to the New York scene by her sister. "As the older sister of a surgical resident in the front lines of the pandemic in New York City, I feel helpless. Every day I operate with a redundant supply of gowns, masks, and gloves while she and her colleagues struggle to gather one complete set of the appropriate personal protective equipment to take care of acutely ill patients swarming the Emergency Department or undergoing emergent intubation (placing a tube into the airway so that a ventilator can 'breathe' for the patient). To make matters worse,

Section Two

residents were expected to financially provide for their own protection. I do my best to spread the word about her fundraiser to purchase more personal protective equipment for the residents in her hospital, but am I doing enough to guarantee her safety? I feel guilty that I cannot protect her and that she does not have what I have. During our daily chats, I can see in her face the fatigue and despair that most of us cannot even imagine. Recently, she shared with me her sadness over the deaths of two young and previously healthy medicine residents (internal medicine trainees), who contracted COVID-19. They remained in the ICU and succumbed, unable to wean from the ventilator. They were my sister's colleagues and friends. To me, they could have been her. I feel sheltered and forcibly distant from what she and her colleagues were seeing and experiencing every day."

We neurosurgeons were relegated to the ranks of unessential personnel during the COVID-19 pandemic. We are not used to being in this role. We are usually up front leading charges, saving lives and performing heroic operations that make a real difference in people's lives. Not so the days of the pandemic. This can leave us with a sense of uselessness and, to some degree, depression, a sense of despair and, of course, anxiety.

We appeared to be consumed with the current stressors, as they affected us directly from the heat of battle. What about the long term? How do we recover from the pandemic? What challenges will we face? A sixth-year neurosurgery resident at the Cleveland Clinic at the time brought up another stressor: job availability. "In this 'new normal' state of affairs, I am incredibly anxious about the prospect finding it difficult to enter the job market as an academic neurosurgical oncologist. The senior residents (like myself), who are going to be graduating in the next year or two, will likely compete with each other for a limited number of job opportunities brought about by a 'new normal' resulting from the pandemic. It is likely that no number of publications, references, and prior funding successes will be enough to entice a neurosurgery department to offer me a staff position. This is of particular concern if I were to require research start-up funding in the 'new normal' resource stressed environment. Hospitals will likely be on hiring freezes and may even be looking to cull the number of neurosurgeons on staff. No one has any idea of what the neurosurgical job market will look like as we move forward with the pandemic behind us. The 'new normal,' and what

Section Two

it will bring to the table, terrifies me. It, in fact, terrifies me more than the anxiety associated with the fear of COVID-19- related death."

So, how does one manage emotions and feelings, let alone the feelings and emotions of trainees in circumstances such as the COVID-19 pandemic? Many of us lived in some sort of isolation during the pandemic, with time to think and escalate the perceived magnitude of the situation in our own minds. As we all know, our minds, if allowed to "run wild," can play cruel tricks on our psyche. To answer my question, I have a three-word answer: "TALK and LISTEN." We can have virtual meetings to talk over our anxieties, fears, and feelings of guilt, as we do at the Cleveland Clinic. We then can lean on each other. We listen to each other. We should honestly and openly discuss our feelings and emotions. Talking, and perhaps more importantly listening, is most certainly cathartic. It provides each of us with insight into our own emotions and, in turn, can help each of us help each other.

Obviously, much has unfolded since the surge associated with the pandemic in early 2020. Some fears dissipated, while others escalated. Nevertheless, we can learn from the past and use what we learned to make the future better.

Section Two

Essay 13
Mindfulness

This article was republished in WORLD NEUROSURGERY and again here, with permission, from the *AANS Neurosurgeon:* (*https://aansneurosurgeon.org/features/the-mindful-neurosurgeon-and-the-art-of-doing-whats-right/*).

I feel that the message is appropriate for this venue. Hence, I am re-publishing with the hopes of reaching an even wider international audience of physicians and non-physicians alike. I have left this primarily as originally published; ie, for neurosurgeons.. Hopefully, it will provide food for thought for neurosurgeons and non-neurosurgeons alike.

The Mindful Neurosurgeon and the Art of Doing What's Right

Being a mindful neurosurgeon is a lofty and on the surface a seemingly complex goal, indeed. Over a decade ago, I was in the audience for a lecture on spine surgery at a national meeting. The lecture hall was packed and each person in the audience had access to an audience-response system. The speaker presented a case and asked the simple question "Would you recommend surgery for the patient just presented?" Roughly 80% answered in the affirmative. Subsequently, he asked the question "Would you undergo this operation yourself?" Roughly 80% answered in the negative. This dichotomy is damning for our profession. Simply put, this is a violation of the *Golden Rule*—do unto others as you would have done unto yourself. Mindfulness was not featured in the lecture hall that day. I am not sure of the right thing to do in that case, but I am certain that the majority of the surgeons in the room, at least during the timeframe encompassing the lecture, were not mindful. They were not focused on the *Golden Rule*.

A Calling

Many factors have driven neurosurgeons to who they become as physicians. These include personal gratification, professional advancement and monetary gain. But, the

Section Two

aforementioned factors are more or less mechanical and are representative of what most people associate with the advantages associated with their job. Paul Kalanithi, in his riveting book *When Breath Becomes Air*,[1] addresses this very point in discussing the notion that physicians should be or become selfless, i.e., place our patients' interests above our own. He then makes a clear separation between a job and a calling. As an aside, this passage and book are referenced multiple times elsewhere in this book.

"Indeed, this is how 99 percent of people select their jobs: pay, work environment, hours. But that's the point. Putting lifestyle first is how you find a job—not a calling."

The mindful neurosurgeon has mastered the art of doing what's right. The mindful neurosurgeon does not look at a job from the perspective of the job being a commodity generator, but from the perspective of the job being a calling.

Becoming a Mindful Leader

We neurosurgeons are all leaders and should act accordingly. Good leaders are selfless. They are egalitarian. They have visions and possess self-direction as well as the ability to motivate. They are socially and self-aware. In other words, they are mindful of themselves and those with whom they interact. They have a worldview that causes them to do what is right.

Good, mindful leaders guide patients to better places. They are concerned much more about doing what's right than they are about revenue generation or academic advancement. They focus on the good they do (value-based care), not on how much they do (volume-based care).

Truly mindful leaders also perpetually reflect. They honestly assess themselves and their own actions. They are very critical of their own results. They strive for honesty. The words of Sir William Osler resonate here (from *The Student Life*, 1905 and referenced several times elsewhere in this book):

> *Begin early to make a threefold category—clear cases, doubtful cases, mistakes. And learn to play the game fair. No self-deception. No shrinking from the truth. Mercy and consideration for the other man. But none for yourself, upon whom you have to keep an incessant watch....*

Section Two

It is only by getting your cases grouped in this way that you can make any real progress in your education; only in this way can you gain wisdom from experience.[2]

Finally, and most importantly, mindful leaders are empathic. Empathy has two components: caring and showing that care. Most people care. Most neurosurgeons care about people, results and interpersonal interactions. All of us, however, occasionally fail to express the fact that we care. Being aware of oneself and how to project in conversation and action is a truly difficult task. Self-awareness is integrally woven in with social-awareness (the ability to understand and respond to the needs of others). These terms can be thought of in the context of how we project ourselves, versus how we perceive and respond to the needs of others.[3] Bottom line, we need to remain mindful and considerate.

The Truly Mindful Neurosurgeon

Hence, the mindful neurosurgeon is an empathic leader who values doing what is right over all else and approaches his/her career as a calling. Sounds simple, but it is oh so difficult to achieve. Remembering the words of Osler may serve us all well as we strive to achieve the pinnacle of mindfulness. Doing all these things may appear difficult or even impossible at first, but that can become a labor of love with nurturing and work. Then, it feeds on itself! When we do what is right, we get good results. Good outcomes result in job satisfaction and fulfillment. Satisfaction and fulfillment, in turn, result in happiness. A happy surgeon is an effective and productive surgeon. This all boils down to "doing what's right"!

Endnotes

1. Kalanithi, P. (2019). *When Breath Becomes Air*. Random House, USA.
2. Osler, W. (1905). *The Student Life: A Farewell Address to Canadian and American Medical Students*. Publisher not identified.

Section Two

Essay 14
Thank You, Dr. Xue

Sometimes it is appropriate to "bend or break the rules." The case of Drs. Fuqiang Xi and Jijiao Xue exemplifies such. Drs. Xi and Xue submitted a manuscript to **World Neurosurgery** in May 2019. After completing the peer review process, the manuscript was accepted for publication in July 2019. Repeated attempts to contact the authors to finalize the page proofs, such as the following, failed:

> *I recently contacted you regarding outstanding corrections for the above referenced article but have not yet received a reply. As we have not received a response from you for quite some time we shall proceed to withdraw your article from production 30 days from the date of this email unless we hear back from you within that time. Please kindly note that if your article is withdrawn and you still wish for it to be published you will need to start the submission process again and resubmit via the editorial system for peer review. In order for your paper not be withdrawn please get in touch as soon as possible.*

After no response was received from multiple similar emails, the below letter was sent:

> *Dear Authors: Just a gentle reminder on my email below.* **We shall proceed to withdraw your paper by the end of this week 2nd April**, *unless we hear back from you regarding your proof corrections.*

There was no response and the article was withdrawn from production in early April 2020. Then, after months went by, we at **WORLD NEUROSURGERY** received the following from Dr. Xue on July 3, 2020:

Section Two

Dear editor,

Thank you for your email. I apologize for my late response. From beginning of August in 2019, I participated in a project aimed to raise the medical level in poor counties, and we need to stay there for half a year. Where I stayed is a remote village, and we cannot use the web, so we cannot check my email box. After we came back from the village, the COVID-19 happened in China, and I need to face the epidemic situation with my colleagues until recent days.

I do not have time to check my email box until now and find the email of proof. I know that it's maybe late to respond your email, and I saw that my manuscript has been withdrawn. There are lots of things happened in these days and I hope you can give me another opportunity to correct my proof and re-press it. When I submitted the manuscript, editors and reviewers are showed their interests in my paper, and I hope to publish my article in **World Neurosurgery** *so much.*

I find that the link of proof is still work, may I use the link to correct proof? Once again, I apologize for any inconvenience caused by my late response, and I will be most grateful if you could offer us a second opportunity.

With kind regards,
Yours sincerely,
Jijiao Xue

We at **WORLD NEUROSURGERY** had already withdrawn the manuscript. Normally we would ask for a resubmission and to start the peer review process over, which would add months to the publication process. But this was a special and unique case, and my response internally at **WORLD NEUROSURGERY** reflected such:

> I think we should reprocess if we can.
> This neurosurgeon is doing what more folks should do on the global neurosurgery platform.

Section Two

He should not be punished for it.
It's kind of a heartwarming story.

And reprocess we did. It was released online on July 25, 2020, and the page proofs have since been finalized.

The manuscript was published: *https://doi.org/10.1016/j.wneu.2020.07.156*.

Let us pause, step back a bit and think about what Dr. Xue and team did for neurosurgery and for mankind. It is not such a big deal that we broke the rule regarding withdrawal, essentially on a compassionate basis—i.e., treat the good guys well. It is a big deal, though, that Dr. Xue and team dedicated so much of their life (greater than a half-year) and then came back only to face another disaster (COVID-19).

We must honor and respect those who give so much and ask for so little in return. In this case, the least we can do is facilitate dissemination of information and promote the neurosurgery academic mission.

This scenario penetrates to the heart of what **WORLD NEUROSURGERY** is all about. Our goal is not to have the highest impact factor and not necessarily to publish the most sophisticated scientific manuscripts. Our goal at **WORLD NEUROSURGERY** is to disseminate information, seek low- and medium-income-country neurosurgeons as our prime target for education, promote the academic mission and, finally, honor those who serve and particularly those who have sacrificed.

For those unfamiliar with medicine and academic publications, impact factor is a metric that addresses the frequency of citations for articles published in the journal. In a way, impact factor provides an assessment of academic profile, but not necessarily value to the readership. **WORLD NEUROSURGERY** aims to provide content for ALL neurosurgeons—particularly low- and medium-income regions of the world.

So, thank you, Dr. Xue, for all you do—from your high-level academic publications to your sacrifices aimed at making this world a better place in which to live.

Section Two

Essay 15

Empowerment

Empowerment: the authority or power given to someone to do something. The process of becoming stronger and more confident.

Empowerment, if considered from the perspective of the raw definition, does not appear to be a term of great significance. "The authority or power given to someone to do something" is routine in the hierarchy of the workplace, organizations, countries, and in life in general. "The process of becoming stronger and more confident," however, gives us a hint regarding the importance of empowerment and, perhaps more importantly, on being or becoming empowered. Becoming strong and confident is, in large part, the foundation for growth and maturation process that is integral to becoming successful adults, leaders, and compassionate and empathic human beings.

Hence, I argue that the word empowerment is a term that is associated with greater significance than that which immediately appears at the outset. Empowerment is what we do when we give our children the confidence and skills to ride a bicycle. Empowerment is what a manager does when assigning important jobs to employees. The effective manager "sees" the employee maturing with each incrementally important and perhaps increasingly difficult assigned task. The employee, because he or she has been bestowed with the honor (of sorts) associated with the obvious growing confidence that the manager has demonstrated, leads the employee to become more confident. This, in turn, fosters leadership skills (leadership: the art of causing others to do something they otherwise would not have done). The process becomes iterative and an ongoing productive relationship between the manager and the employee grows.

From a physician's perspective, the empowerment of associates (i.e., nurses, technicians, clerks, advanced practice providers, and others) is critical to the development and nurturing of a highly skilled and functional team. Confidence in each member of the team in each other and with themselves is a critical component of effective

Section Two

teams. Each member of the team has been empowered to function at a high level. In turn, each member empowers other team members to do the same.

Let us turn to the physician-patient relationship. It is well known that patients, when given treatment option choices, are much more likely to comply with the treatment option they chose, when compared to a treatment option dictated by the physician. The physician, in this patient-choice scenario, is empowering the patient to help guide his or her own care. The physician, by giving the patient a treatment goal as a target, may then allow the patient to craft a pathway to that goal. Physicians, however, are often rigid regarding the pathway to the treatment goal choice, thereby not allowing the patient to participate in the decision-making process. This is a paternalistic approach, if you will. In this case, the physician has not empowered the patient, and hence the patient will be less likely to be compliant.

Regardless of the scenario (i.e., parent-child, spouse-spouse, physician-patient, manager-employee, etc.), the empowerment of others is a critical key to the fostering of productive and meaningful relationships. So, the term empowerment and the act of being empowered are so much more important than the raw definition implies. We all need to place the empowerment of others as a top-level priority regarding interpersonal communication and the assignment of responsibilities. We should also perpetually seek to earn the privilege of being empowered by demonstrating that we deserve the trust of others. Bottom line: Think empowerment, empower others, and seek to become deserving of being empowered.

Section Two

Essay 16
The Imposter Syndrome

The Imposter Syndrome – Definitions:

"The belief that one is incompetent in their field, that others have more knowledge or skills than they do in a certain area, or that their accomplishments are due to luck, chance, or even their appearance, and has little to do with their own efforts or hard work."
– Sydney Hausberger [1]

"In simplified terms: you feel like you're a fraud, you don't deserve your success, and that you'll eventually be exposed as a fraud."
–Tim Harrison [2]

The imposter syndrome has gotten a lot of press recently, predominantly due to the fact that the majority of us are victims of the syndrome to one degree or another.[3] It was originally studied in high-achieving women with self-doubt who harbored the feeling that they were frauds by Pauline Clance and Suzanne Imes in 1978.[4] They coined the term "imposter phenomenon" and observed it in women. It is now recognized to be common in both women and men.

The term "imposter syndrome" has been studied and recognized increasingly over the years. But, what is it exactly and why do some people seem to identify with it? Imposter syndrome refers to the belief that one is incompetent in their field, that others have more knowledge or skills than they do in a certain area, or that their accomplishments are due to luck, chance, or even their appearance, and has little to do with their own efforts or hard work. These individuals are typically high-achievers and feel this way despite having previous experiences of success. In addition, they are unable to internalize their accomplishments, causing feelings of

Section Two

persistent self-doubt. According to Hausberger,[1] the key features of the imposter syndrome include:

- Being worried that you may appear like a fraud or "imposter" and fear that you will be called out for being "incompetent."
- Thinking that everyone around you is smarter or works harder than you do.
- You do not believe that you are capable of doing things, even if there is evidence that you have succeeded/done well in the past.
- You are self-critical of your work and compare yourself to others.
- You may feel inadequate, do not trust yourself, feel anxious, or lack confidence.

I would guess that neurosurgeons are neither more immune nor more prone to the imposter syndrome. In this regard, they are like all over-achievers. A little self-doubt may be healthy, not unlike the notion that a little over-confidence may be healthy as well. However, the harboring of significant self-doubt can be destructive, as can supreme, unjustified over-confidence, in both neurosurgeons and non-neurosurgeons.

My intent here is to heighten awareness and inform regarding the imposter syndrome. One might ask, how does one manage self-doubt and low confidence? Making a mental "connection" between self-doubt and low confidence with the imposter syndrome is critical. The first and foremost step is to recognize the existence of the imposter syndrome and appreciate that you may be affected; i.e., awareness. For many of those reading this, the notion of imposter syndrome is foreign. The recognition of its existence when present, hence, is imperative. Unhealthy self-doubt, if unrecognized, can decrease performance and be psychologically destructive. Once recognized, the institution of a self-confidence reclamation project is in order—that is, if one is adversely affected by the syndrome. Once the imposter syndrome is recognized as an actual entity as above (Step 1) and one recognizes that they may have the syndrome (Step 2), the next two critical steps, acceptance (Step 3) and the discipline to address the problem (Step 4) are essential for effective management. These four steps represent half the battle.

I am not an expert with the imposter syndrome, nor am I a psychologist or therapist. I have, however, "coached" colleagues who have grappled with self-doubt and diminished self-confidence. Perhaps most importantly and in the spirit of transparency, I believe that I have the syndrome. I am working on it. There is an abundance of self-help literature that, for the most part, is helpful.[1,2] Honing in on self-awareness and social-awareness skills (Section 1, Essay 9) can most certainly help one negotiate this abyss. Obviously, if the problem persists or progresses, professional help may be prudent.

On the flip side of all the aforementioned, a little self-doubt, as previously mentioned, may be used to fuel the motivation required to improve performance.[5] For many imposter syndrome sufferers, self-doubt can lead to overachievement via the extra effort expended to improve meaningful communication with colleagues and to potentially outperform non-imposter colleagues.

Bottom line, think imposter syndrome and self-doubt, and assess whether or not such affects you. If so, deal with it accordingly. It is better to be cognizant of your deficits, so that you can intelligently manage them. It simply makes sense to embrace self-doubt, if possible, and use it, as stated, to fuel improved performance. In my case, I think I am doing such, but I have a long way to go.

Endnotes

1. Hausberger, S. The imposter syndrome; what it is and what you can do about it. *https://sagewellnessctr.org/2021/06/imposter-syndrome-what-it-is-what-you-can-do-about-it/*.
2. Harrison T: Let's See Who You Really Are! Unmasking Imposter Syndrome: *https://www.extremenetworks.com/*.
3. Bravata, D. M.; S. A. Watts; A. L. Keefer; D. K. Madhusudhan; K. T. Taylor; D. M. Clark; and H. K. Hagg (2020). Prevalence, predictors, and treatment of impostor syndrome: a systematic review. *Journal of General Internal Medicine,* 35(4), 1252-1275. *https://doi.org/10.1007/s11606-019-05364-1*.
4. Clance, P. R., and S. A. Imes (1978). The imposter phenomenon in high achieving women: Dynamics and therapeutic intervention. *Psychotherapy: Theory, Research & Practice,* 15(3), 241–247. *https://doi.org/10.1037/h0086006*.
5. Rubinstein P: The Hidden Upside of the Imposter Syndrome. *https://www.bbc.com/worklife/article/20210315-the-hidden-upside-of-imposter-syndrome*.

Section Two

Essay 17
Hello, How Are You?

About seven or eight years ago, my wife Mary and I were vacationing in Niagara by the Lake in beautiful southern Ontario, Canada. As we strolled along the streets of this quaint little town, we came across a coffee shop. On the sidewalk in front of the coffee shop a sign read as follows:

Coffee - $5
Coffee—with a "Hello" - $2
Coffee—with a "Hello, how are you?" - $1

To this day, I kick myself for not taking a photograph of the sign. Regardless, the imagery and relevance of the sign have stuck with me over the years. How delightfully simple, and yet both complex and beautifully genuine, are these words! They are simple by virtue of the few words employed to convey a message and beautifully genuine because of the refreshing message conveyed. They are also complex by virtue of the engagement of two individuals who are sharing a brief empathic moment—if you will, a brief, genuine exchange of kindness and an expression of concern for another.

The words "Hello, how are you?" can be used to send a complex message that, as stated, is one of genuine concern and compassion. The complexity is amplified by the intricacies associated with being "in the moment" with another human being, even if the "moment" is brief. The same words, however, and unfortunately, are often uttered reflexively and without much forethought or afterthought regarding intent or concern for the other participant(s) in the conversation. The latter, in a sense, represents a feeble attempt to be politely conversational—but alas, without significant meaning or substance and without a true connection between the participants. The two individuals in this case are most certainly not "in the moment" with each other.

Section Two

So, what differentiates the impact of two utterances of "Hello, how are you?" What differentiates a brief exchange of words in which the same words convey very different messages? The art of listening plays a pivotal role here. Listening and genuinely responding to the question allows one to meaningfully engage another "in the moment." "I am so happy that you are having a good day—so am I...."

Conversely, if one utters the "Hello, how are you?" question, buys the coffee, does not listen to the response, and simply moves on, the interaction is rendered meaningless. Listening and responding accordingly and empathically may be all it takes to make someone smile. It can even lead to further and even more meaningful conversation. You will never know what will transpire unless you try.

I guess my message here can be distilled into the following: When confronting another human being, use the words "Hello, how are you?" frequently. Most importantly, though, is what you do next. Listen. No, carefully listen to the response. And, then, act accordingly by being "in the moment." More than likely you will, at the very least, cause someone to smile. ☺

Section Two

Essay 18
The Dunning-Kruger Effect

Dunning-Krueger effect:
A hypothetical cognitive bias stating that people with low ability at a task overestimate their own ability, and that people with high ability at a task underestimate their own ability.
(Definition from Wikipedia)

The *Dunning-Kruger Effect* has two components, or poles, if you will. One is manifested by an overestimation of competence and the other by an underestimation of competence. The *Dunning-Kruger Effect* occurs when an individual's suboptimal foundation of knowledge and/or skill causes him/her to overestimate his/her own competence. By contrast, this effect also occurs in those who excel regarding knowledge and/or skill to think a task is simple for everyone. This causes the individual to underestimate their relative abilities. I covered the latter (imposter syndrome) in Section 2, Essay 16. I will now focus on the overestimation of competence in this chapter.

The over-estimation of one's own competence is common. Such may be a manifestation, or a result of, denial. Such denial, in turn, results from suboptimal self- and social-awareness. This cognitive bias, which is a systematic pattern of deviation from the norm, represents a lapse of rationality in judgment.[1] In Section 1, Essay 9, I discussed self- and social-awareness. Both are relevant here. Self awareness is an awareness of one's own personality or individuality, whereas social awareness is the ability to comprehend and appropriately react to both broad problems of society and interpersonal struggles.

Social- and self awareness are very different but are essentially inextricably linked, as previously stated. Asking oneself the question *"How am I coming across?"* and exercising the use of the "social etiquette filter" so that socially inappropriate responses are internalized, and socially appropriate responses are externalized, work hand in hand to help us become more effective communicators and, in fact, empathy is manifested by expressing the fact that we care (empathy). Although self awareness plays a dominant role in this (expression of the fact that we care, i.e., empathy), social awareness plays an accompanying synergistic role. This is much like the way that yin and yang complement each other. Social- and self-awareness skillsets address the task of expressing the fact that one cares from both poles of the task at hand—one by asking oneself, *"How am I coming across?"* and the other by employing the "social etiquette filter" that separates the socially unacceptable from the acceptable. With practice, both can be developed and nurtured.

Each of us creates our own "subjective reality," much of which is dictated by our grasp of our own social- and self-awareness. For those of us who have the imposter syndrome, our own "subjective reality" may be channeled in such a manner that we work harder and, in fact, over-achieve. The opposite pole of the *Dunning Krueger effect*, however, is more harmful, with very little, if any, advantage, or up-side. For those of us without a robust "social etiquette filter," an inability or unwillingness to practice social- and self awareness skills leads to a persona that others can identify as boisterous, egocentric, and over-confident. Being of high confidence and low ability is a very socially dangerous place to be.

So, let us all work on our social- and self-awareness skillsets by focusing on questions such as *"How am I coming across?"* and *"Am I really that good?"* Perpetually posing such questions to ourselves, and forcing ourselves to honestly answer them, will help each of us become a better person who is appropriately appreciated by peers and friends.

Endnote

1. Haselton, M. G.; D. Nettle; and P. W. Andrews. The evolution of cognitive bias. In Buss DM (ed.). *The Handbook of Evolutionary Psychology.* Hoboken, NJ, US: John Wiley and Sons, Inc., pp. 724-726, 2005.

Section Two

Essay 19
Today Will Be a Good Day

In Section 2, Essay 1, entitled *Today Was a Good Day*, I outlined how one can and should derive significant pleasure and fulfillment from helping people negotiate difficult situations and times and by always "doing what's right." Such "management opportunities" often occur randomly. What if there were no "management opportunities" in a given day, or none for a week? In such a situation, how does one feel fulfilled and accomplished? There must be more to "having a good day" than simply doing the right thing and helping people in need. This raises the question, if such "management opportunities" do not arise on any given day, how does one proactively craft a good day?

The proactive crafting of a good day is all about attitude. Beginning the day with the conviction that it WILL be a good day is a great start. If one expects to have a good day, such will likely happen; conversely, it is far too easy for us to feel sorry for ourselves and then transmit negative vibes to friends, family and colleagues. Feeling sorry for ourselves allows us to lower our level of enthusiasm for life in general in our work-related and family-related environment, specifically.

Being positive is so much more fun than being negative. Feeling sorry for oneself lets evil demons enter our psyche. Answering a greeting from another such as "How are you today?" with an "Okay" begs the question "Is something wrong?" One could rather say, "I am great, how are you?" If you say it, you will begin believing it. So, why do we subject ourselves to misery by succumbing to negativity, when all we need to do is be positive? "I am great, how are you?"

We all have haunting prior experiences that plague us by not completely leaving our consciousness. Such prior experiences include a surgical complication and a lawsuit (for physicians), work-related conflict, the loss of a loved one, family strife, the loss of a pet, and on and on. How do we shake these demons that most certainly contribute to a negative attitude? We all have them. Some of us deal effectively with them, while others struggle.

Section Two

What can those who struggle here learn from those who do not? Let me emphasize up front that the inability to keep the demons at bay for a physician may be a manifestation of simply not caring -"I do not care that my patient had a complication." Such is ego-centric and selfish. It is not acceptable and is not discussed further here. We, hence, will focus on legitimate demon management for physicians and non-physicians alike.

Looking at this another way, why do some keep the demons in front of them, thus not allowing them to see past the demons without the demons entering their consciousness, while others keep the demons off to the side, say over their shoulder, thus allowing for a clear view ahead, by relegating the demons to a place where they do not perpetually enter the consciousness of the individual and do not obstruct the view ahead?

I personally struggle with the demons. I seem to worry excessively about multiple issues, at least according to my wife, Mary. I perseverate regarding the aforementioned issues, and hence, keep the demons in front of me so that they "block my clear vision" looking forward, while at the same time gaining access to my consciousness. Mary, on the other hand, does not struggle with the demons to the extent that I do. She keeps them out of view and out of mind. What can I learn from her? After further scrutiny, I believe that Mary believes the following:

1. "Relax, it will be all right"; i.e., do not worry.
2. "I will do it later"—an acceptable strategy, compared to having to do everything now.
3. Keep the mind busy with useful and purposeful thoughts—thus dispersing and seeing past the demons.
4. "Worry when there is something truly worth fretting over; and do not worry about the small stuff."
5. Think about moving forward and strategies to succeed. Do not dwell on the past, for it cannot be changed.

Please keep in mind that worrying and fretting over the big and small stuff is the strategy that many have used to achieve success in their field. My bottom line 'take'

Section Two

here is that I need to learn from Mary, but not give up the tools that helped me achieve whatever it is I have achieved. I will work harder at removing the demons from my view ahead to a place where they become a minor occasional annoyance, but not a horrible and pathological distraction. I, perhaps, need to take a little more of a relaxed attitude to many of my trials and tribulations. Perhaps I should selectively do some things later, rather than now. Procrastination in moderation may not be so bad. I should focus on what I can change and not on things I cannot. Finally, I should choose my battles by purposefully worrying about things that are real problems and worthy of a good worry.

By such compartmentalization and selectively focusing on altering the way we deal with stressors seems to be the key here. Moving forward, I will try to be a little more like Mary; worry less and procrastinate a bit more. ☺

Section Two

Essay 20
Opportunity

Opportunity: a set of circumstances that makes it possible to do something
– Oxford Languages

"Chance favors the prepared mind."
– Louis Pasteur

"When opportunity knocks, open the door."
–Multiple authors

"When opportunity knocks, it's too late to prepare."
–John Wooden

(An American basketball coach and player. He won ten National Collegiate Athletic Association (NCAA) national championships in a twelve-year period as head coach for the UCLA Bruins men's basketball team, including a record seven in a row. No other team has won more than four in a row in Division I college men's or women's basketball championships. Within this period, his teams won an NCAA men's basketball record 88 consecutive games.)

Discoveries, innovations, success at work, success in sports, and success in life revolve around opportunities. The presence of opportunities, the recognition of such opportunities, and the taking advantage of said opportunities all play a role in the achievement of success. The definition of opportunity (a set of circumstances that makes it possible to do something) is simple enough, but the act of capitalizing on an opportunity may be another story.

Let us start with the presentation of opportunities. Leaders in war and peace are borne from the presentation of an opportunity. There are likely hundreds or even

Section Two

thousands of individuals with the leadership skills on par with Winston Churchill. We do not know most of them, though, because opportunity was not presented to them. Mr. Churchill, however, saw opportunity and seized the moment. He, and others, led Great Britain and the free world to victory in World War II. He saw opportunity and assembled the resources to take advantage of it *("When opportunity knocks, open the door")*.

Mr. Churchill recognized the opportunities presented to him, but he did much, much more. First, as stated, he recognized the opportunities. How many "unseen" opportunities are routinely presented to each of us, perhaps daily? Likely, many/most are missed. Keeping a keen eye for opportunity identification is critical, and the subsequent taking advantage of the presented opportunity is paramount. Louis Pasteur's statement *"Chance favors the prepared mind"* is oh so appropriate here. Preparing the mind to be ready to "see" and to be ready and prepared to deal with the presented opportunity is critical. This brings us to the last quote by John Wooden at the top of this article: *"When opportunity knocks, it's too late to prepare."* When opportunity presents itself, there often is no time to prepare for the unique set of circumstances. Thus, a calculated and accurate reaction/action is required. Such can only be achieved by preemptive preparation.

Airline pilots are exposed to many critical scenario simulations in their training that prepares them, in advance, for potential disaster mitigation. In this case the opportunity presents as "an opportunity" to prevent disaster. Due to the training, the new and challenging situation has been "seen" and "dealt with" before during the simulations. On January 15, 2009, US Airways Flight 1549, on a flight from LaGuardia Airport in New York City to Charlotte, North Carolina, struck a flock of birds shortly after takeoff. This resulted in the loss of engine power. The pilots (Chesley "Sully" Sullenberger and Jeffrey Skiles) were unable to reach an airport for an emergency landing due to their low altitude. Hence, they glided the plane to a "ditching" in the Hudson River off Midtown Manhattan. All 155 people on board were rescued by nearby boats, with only a few serious injuries.

This is a great story, but it is even a better lesson. Preemptive preparation for expected and unexpected situations is the key. The pilot's reactions and actions with

Section Two

Flight 1549 saved lives, many lives. Just imagine how many similar situations in all fields did not go so well. John Wooden's statement, *"When opportunity knocks, it's too late to prepare,"* so aptly implies the need for preemptive preparation. That's how one wins multiple championships and safely lands an impaired airplane. It is also how surgeons salvage unexpected intraoperative findings or events.

So, no matter what your profession or where your aims in life guide you, try as best you can, to prepare for the unexpected. Be ready with a "plan B." "Plan A" does not always work the way you had anticipated.

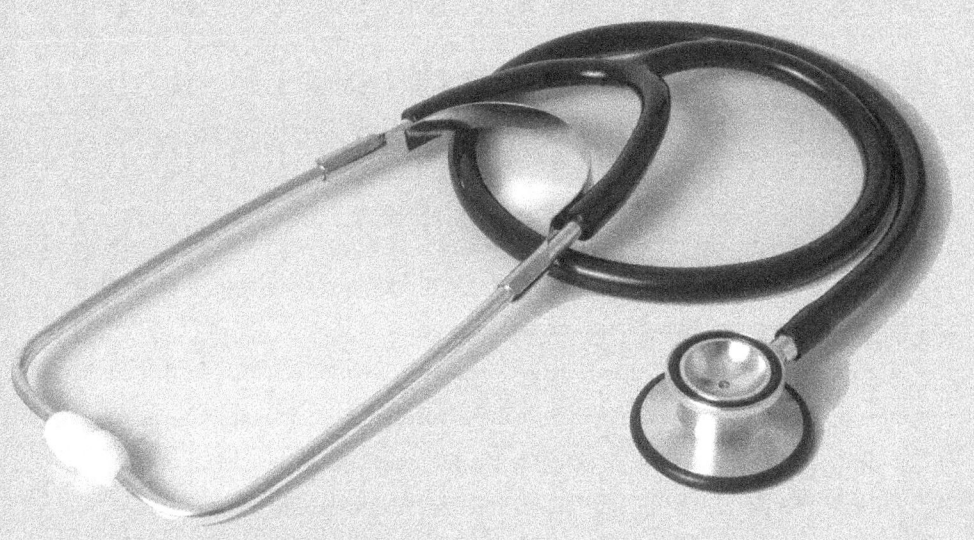

SECTION THREE: INTRODUCTION

Lessons from the Medical Arena

The prior two sections have focused on lessons regarding effective communication and fulfillment. The chapters in this section (Section 3) focus on specific interactions between neurosurgeons and patients and/or specific processes that affect neurosurgeons and that can be repurposed into lessons for all. The chapters that follow are "heavier" and more difficult to "digest" for the lay person. Regardless, give them a whirl. There are many messages here.

Section Three

Essay 1

Bias, Therapeutic Illusion and the Illusion of Control

In the March 31, 2016, issue of the *New England Journal of Medicine,* David Casarett provided a very timely and much-needed perspective on medical decision making and the factors that cause physicians to, at times, make unwise decisions.[1] In this dissertation, he states, "The outcome of virtually all medical decisions is at least partly outside the physician's control, and random chance can encourage physicians to embrace mistaken beliefs about causality." He also refers to confirmation bias: "Once a treatment is under way, physicians (and patients) tend to look for evidence that it is having some kind of positive effect." He emphasizes using two heuristics—i.e., rules of thumb—when making decisions based on "data" and observations:

1. "Before you conclude that a treatment was effective, look for other explanations."
2. "If you see evidence of success, look for evidence of failure."

First, for the non-medical, lay public readers, this discussion most certainly makes one uneasy. It implies that doctors aren't what they were thought to be—i.e., scholars, always with the "right answer." Doctors are human and, hence, fall into the same traps as all other humans when assessing data. The concepts presented here are not new concepts, but Casarett brings them to our attention at an opportune time. All doctors are guilty of succumbing to both the therapeutic illusion and the illusion of control. They, however, seldom use the aforementioned heuristics. Such increases cost and perhaps risks decreasing the efficacy and safety of care. Unfortunately, these decision-making foibles spill over into the publication arena. Both the therapeutic illusion and the illusion of control allow bias to adversely affect study design and, hence, publication validity (also disconcerting for the non-medical lay public). There exist mounting

Section Three

concerns regarding the publication of false findings.[2] We are all prone to being victimized by bias, whether medical or non-medical.

Medical journals and publications are increasingly on alert to detect bias and false and misleading findings. This will hopefully increase the validity of the published literature. We all must remain cognizant of our tendencies to fall prey to the therapeutic illusion and the illusion of control, because of bias and/or misguided enthusiasm regarding a treatment or strategy. Self-discipline and honest assessment of self and others is mandatory here.

Endnotes

1. Casarett, D. The Science of Choosing Wisely - Overcoming the Therapeutic Illusion. N Engl J Med, 2016 (374:1203-120).
2. Ioannidis, JPA (2005). Why most published research findings are false. PLoS Med 2(8): e124.

Section Three

Essay 2

Managing Illness

The unspoken mission of neurosurgeons is to treat disease by managing illness. The patient's disease is the "enemy" of the care providers (i.e. physicians, nurses, etc.) and the patient and the patient's family. The team is composed of the surgeon, other patient care providers, the patient and relevant family, and friends. This team utilizes a variety of resources and tools to "fight" the "enemy," e.g., by resecting a brain tumor and the provision of postoperative care. In most circumstances, the treatment of the disease is the simple part. Managing the illness, however, often presents a challenge of a much higher order.

Managing illness is centered about understanding and dealing with the impact of the disease (e.g., brain tumor) on the patient, family and friends from a psychosocial and perhaps a financial perspective. Such a holistic approach to disease and illness not only deals with the "bio-"component of the bio-psychosocial theory of disease, but it also deals with the psychosocial component as well—with an emphasis on the latter.

Managing illness, from the healthcare provider's perspective, involves the establishment of mutual respect, usually via the creation of an emotional connection. The latter is nurtured by developing lines of communication that are based on a genuine interest in each other, with the mutual goal of a shared commitment to physical and mental health. This psychosocial approach to the deliverance of healthcare may not always be achieved. The patient with a brain tumor may not harbor an adequate grasp of the very complex nature of his/her disease. In addition, such a patient is obligatorily under an immense amount of stress. Such a patient or his/her family and friends may manifest their stress by expressing anger, which may be compounded by their suboptimal comprehension of the complexities of their condition. Such a patient can be challenging, thus potentially placing the physician/patient relationship in peril.

Physicians must remember that not all patients will become their friends, nor will the physician and patient agree on everything. Nevertheless, the physician must

Section Three

remain vigilant regarding the assurance that the patient, family and friends are adequately informed and educated so that appropriate decisions are made, and compliance is optimized. The physician must establish and maintain boundaries (e.g., restrictions on duration of postoperative narcotic prescriptions, etc.). By the way, so should the patient. The physician must strive to guide the patient to a better place. The patient should be working with the physician in this regard. The physician should remember that he/she is a leader, and that leadership is the art of causing others to deliberately create a result that otherwise would not have happened (see Section 1, Essay 4).

I would be remiss here if I did not address the most important communication tool of all: empathy (see Section 1, Essay 1). Being empathic is, without question, the most effective means of achieving the aforementioned goals and for appropriately managing illness. Such is so very simple, yet all too often neglected. All we need to do is express the fact that we care. PERPETUALLY expressing the fact that we care should be our goal with all of our communications. We must aggressively strive to NEVER let our guard down in moments of lapsed self-awareness. ALL OF US can do better here. Physicians can, indeed, improve their illness management skills, but in order to do such they must work at it. Such skills can be improved with practice.

So, let us all make empathy and empathic communication a goal and, in fact, a priority. Let us do such by working at it!!!

Section Three

Essay 3

The Art of Surgery

"Have we strayed too far?"

In a way, the act of surgery is an art form. The surgeon carves, manipulates, and caresses delicate tissue and it's often difficult to penetrate protective coverings to achieve a predetermined goal—much as a sculptor carves, manipulates and caresses the often delicate and sometimes seemingly impenetrable amorphous rock that will be, in the end, an "object of beauty." Both the surgeon and the sculptor look to create their respective "objects of beauty," and both are artists. With the surgeon, this may be associated with a beautiful dissection and good clinical result. With the sculptor, the resulting object of beauty stands on its own to be judged and to define the degree of success for which the sculptor strives.

With this essay, I will deviate a bit from the conventional writing style used elsewhere in this book. I am going to tell a medical story and, in so doing, pay homage to a pioneer neurosurgeon, Don Prolo. Don Prolo, and those who preceded him in the spine fusion domain, most notably Ralph Cloward, stand apart from many spine surgeons—in that they used very few resources to create great results. This is much like the sculptor who uses his bare hands and a few tools to create a "thing of beauty." In the early days of the posterior lumbar interbody fusion (PLIF) operation (a highly technical operation in which bone grafts were placed between vertebrae), surgeons like Cloward and Prolo developed and evolved the PLIF technique out of necessity. Stability of the spine, in those days, could only be achieved by creative strategies—such as carefully prepared cadaveric bone grafts and meticulous interbody graft bed preparation. Such required, in a sense, master-craftsmen—not unlike the skills required of a master cabinet maker. The "mother of necessity" dictated such to find consistent success, as demonstrated by Prolo et al in this issue ("Un-instrumented Posterior Lumbar Interbody Fusion: Have Technological Advances in Stabilizing the Lumbar Spine Truly Improved Outcomes?") This is an article published in **World**

Section Three

Neurosurgery in July 2018. Cloward's and Prolo's careful and strategic creation of an interbody fusion provided stability while leading to a high fusion rate and remarkable clinical success—a success rate that is infrequently achieved these days, in spite of the utilization of far advanced technologies. They accomplished this success by doing more with less, i.e., achieving stability and decompression (relieving pressure on nerves) via carefully planned, skillfully performed surgery, and without the use of modern stabilization techniques.

Nowadays, spine surgery techniques have devolved from this "art form" to a reliance on technologies that facilitate fusion and decompression of the spine in such a way that surgical skill is often replaced by a reliance on expensive assistive technologies. No longer is the artful surgeon required. The surgery can now be completed with the assistance of image guidance technologies (computer-assisted image guidance), a variety of anchors and cages (a variety of spinal implants), and biologics (agents that are alleged to stimulate bone fusion, but not without risk) that facilitate fusion in order to provide an advantage for the surgeon and the patient. This is good in a way, but I must ask the question: "Have we strayed too far from the art of surgery?" The assistive gadgets and gizmos come at a very high price—a price that we may not be able to afford, as the cost of medical care in the United States and is approaching 20% of the gross domestic product. In addition, these technologies have permitted the average surgeon to achieve the same results as a much more accomplished surgeon (artist), while creating a situation that facilitates the employment of a lower threshold for the performance of surgery. It, in fact, goes without saying that the rate of surgery for pain of spinal origin is rapidly increasing, without the demonstration of a correlative success. Coutinho, in his invited perspective (in ***World Neurosurgery***) on this subject (Prolo's manuscript), concludes with the following thought-provoking and insightful commentary: "Being an observational case series, the article presented by Prolo et al. has a low level of evidence. Undeniably, multi-centric, controlled, and randomized trials showing higher levels of evidence are necessary in order to accept the conclusions presented in this article. Nevertheless, the study is large and shows long-term follow up of patients who underwent PLIF without instrumentation. It will hopefully incite the revision of some of our current paradigms involving lumbar fusion surgery, and

Section Three

instigate discussion on whether cheaper, simpler, and safer techniques may once again be considered as good options for lumbar arthrodesis (fusion)."

Akhavan-Sigari et al, in their invited perspective on Prolo et al's paper, appropriately echo the comments of Coutinho by pointing out that "Despite a large number of publications of outcomes after spinal fusion surgery, there is still no consensus on the relative efficacy of the several different fusion techniques." They also emphasize that "iliac crest bone graft versus other fusion methods remains an area of clinical equipoise (a measure of uncertainty regarding the right thing to do), and further investigations on this topic with prospective randomized trials is warranted."

We have come so far, yet we still do not know the truth regarding optimal strategies for spine care and, for that matter, much of non-spine medical problems—and perhaps we never will. One thing is for certain: We must control costs while providing value in the form of quality outcomes. Perhaps by refocusing on the "art of surgery" while more cautiously embracing new and expensive technologies, we can achieve better results with less expense by carving, manipulating and caressing the spine and its sensitive neural contents—much like the sculptor. Have we strayed too far? In my opinion, we have. The ultimate answer to this question should be individualized, however. Such is up to each surgeon and, for that matter, the patients as well, to decide.

Bottom line here, the lay person should be aware of the uncertainties in medicine, which includes the over-reliance on technology. The lay public and physicians of all specialties must share and discuss these uncertainties so that more effective and less costly treatments are provided by master physicians.

Section Three

Essay 4
Process vs Conclusion-Based Research: Why Should We Care?

"There are three kinds of lies: Lies, damned lies, and statistics."
– Mark Twain;
also attributed to Benjamin Disraeli and Charles Wentworth Dilke

"There are three kinds of lies: Lies, damned lies, and statistics" is an often quoted sarcastic "take" on modern-day research. It seems that one can prove nearly anything one sets out to prove via valid "tried and true" research strategies.

In a 2013 *New England Journal of Medicine* article previously referenced in this book (Section 3, Essay 1), David Casarett discussed concepts that particularly pertain, and are very relevant, to the modern-day surgical literature.[1] In this article, Casarett described the *Therapeutic Illusion*, with which "The outcome of virtually all medical decisions is at least partly outside the physician's control, and random chance can encourage physicians to embrace mistaken beliefs about causality." This leads to *Confirmation Bias*, which may cause a "blind eye" that often leads to the misinterpretation of information. In Casarett's words, "Once a treatment is under way, physicians (and patients) tend to look for evidence that it is having some kind of positive effect." This is as opposed to a truly and honestly objective assessment of the outcomes and findings. Such wishful thinking, and its related skewed interpretation of data and observations, is the essence of *human nature*; i.e, a natural but flawed characteristic of most humans. In his dissertation, Casarett essentially reintroduced concepts conceived by Thomas decades prior (Thomas, K. B. The Consultation and the Therapeutic Illusion. *British Medical Journal*, 1978, 1, 1327-1328).

Casarett's observations, in a way, should cause us to pause, and perhaps to rethink the basis on which surgical decisions are made—most notably, the impact of the surgical literature on the clinical decision-making process—or, for that matter, decision

Section Three

making in general. Our "thinking" may often be flawed, but unfortunately this flawed thinking has traditionally not penetrated our collective cognitive sphere of awareness. As a result, manuscripts that present data that is of questionable validity have been used to create clinical algorithms for care by both surgeons and other consumers of said literature. Many may "feel" that something is awry, but the identification of the associated methodological flaws remains, to them, a mystery.

The literature abounds with conflicting reports involving a singular and distinct subject matter. How can two diverse conclusions be derived, while apparently using similar study designs and methodologies? Such observations have been documented and described by others. For example, the decline effect (the observation that as time passes, study conclusions that seemed based on solid science are gradually proven to be erroneous) has been well described (Lehrer, J. The Truth Wears Off: Is There Something Wrong with the Scientific Method? *Annals of Science,* December 13, 2010) and documented by others, including Ioannidis' introduction of the concept of false findings (Ioannidis, J. P. A. Why Most Published Research Findings Are False (*PLoS Medicine.* Aug. 2005, Volume 2, Issue 8, e124). The cyclical rise and then fall in the rate of utilization of a variety of surgical techniques that were initially enthusiastically embraced, only to subsequently fall out of favor, are manifestations and the end result of false findings and the decline effect. Such a parabolic rise and fall was eloquently described by Scott (Scott, J. W. Scott's Parabola: The Rise and Fall of a Surgical Technique. *British Med J,* 2001; 323:1477). Unfortunately, many suboptimal outcomes and complications, as well as excessive fiscal cost to society result from, and lie in, the wake of the parabolic rise and fall of technology and technique utilization.

Having said all this, you might ask, "What's the point?" What is conclusion-based and process-based research, and by the way, why do I care? First, we should care because we ideally want to determine the truth; hence, an understanding of research paradigms is critical to the achievement of this ideal.

Conclusion-based research can be fundamentally defined as research that is designed *to prove a point.* Significant bias may, unfortunately, befall such research. This is the nature of most prospective clinical trials, particularly randomized prospective surgical trials, with which an attempt to either prove or disprove a hypothesis is undertaken. Involved researchers, either intentionally or unintentionally, seek to *prove a point*, and more often than not achieve their goal.

Conversely, process-based research is designed to determine the truth. An emerging research style termed *exploratory inquiry* exemplifies this process. Such research may, for example, employ registries with which data is collected prospectively and assessed retrospectively. A biased randomization process and study design, hence, is bypassed—as the data is acquired in an unbiased fashion with no preconceived notions. Such facilitates the *finding of the truth*.

Unfortunately, exploratory inquiry (process-based research) is often not funded or is under-funded due to the absence of 'objectivity'. Conclusion-based research (hypothesis testing and driven research) abounds with objectivity and hence is easy to appraise, but the objectivity is often tainted by bias and, hence, flawed (Hauf, C. Why Do Funding Agencies Favor Hypothesis Testing? *Studies in History and Philosophy of Science*, 44 (2013), 363–374).

So, what to do? Well, we can do several things that optimize our assessment of the literature:

1. Be critical of the literature, particularly randomized surgical trials that overtly employ hypothesis testing or that use such without stating. Patients should expect this from their doctors.
2. Remain cognizant of Scott's parabola and scrutinize new technologies or methodologies. They may very well be on the rising part of Scott's curve, only to emerge in the end as a failure. This is unnerving to patients.
3. Challenge new ideas until you are absolutely convinced that they are valid.

Bottom line, remain wary of the human urge to prove a point, because that point may often be wrong! For the non-medical readers, be wary of medical research. Was bias minimized? Were the authors seeking to determine the truth or prove a point? Does the research pass the sniff test? Does it seem reasonable?

Section Three

Essay 5
Who Is Driving the Bus?

Patient compliance is integrally associated with optimized outcomes, regardless of the treatment strategy employed. In physician-patient relationships, a mutual understanding of the problem (e.g., disease) and an agreement on treatment strategy increases the chance of an optimal outcome. Non-compliance, conversely, may often contribute to suboptimal outcomes. Literally translated, if the patient and physician do not see "eye to eye" regarding diagnosis and treatment, suboptimal outcomes will often result. Such results in the patient acting in a manner that is against the wishes of the physician (i.e., non-compliance). There are many contributing factors that are associated with non-compliance. The most common of these, unfortunately, are related to the patient's relative lack of motivation to alter detrimental or even harmful lifestyles. Other factors may be related to lack of adequate patient education regarding the clinical problem at hand. I have made a dangerous assumption here, i.e., that the physician's wishes are appropriate and based on sound judgment and accurate data. Such may occasionally not be the case. Therefore, both parties must be able to justify their position if the need arises.

Altering or eliminating unhealthy habits can be challenging and often unsuccessful when a lack of interest in change, on the part of the patient, prevails. The overtly non-compliant patient may often resist logic and be impervious to active (on the part of the patient) therapies, such as weight loss, cessation of smoking, physical conditioning, aerobic exercises, etc. Such patients often favor passive therapies, such as medications, procedures, and surgery. Such passive therapies do not require effort on the part of the patient. Surgery, if performed in such cases, often fails to achieve the desired outcome, particularly when pain is the underlying clinical complaint.

How can we improve compliance? To simplify, let us focus on the "low-hanging fruit"—i.e., let us focus on patients who are willing to contribute to their own healthcare, but who face barriers to such. The two major barriers in this regard are: 1. in-

Section Three

effective transmission of information from the physician to the patient and 2. the suboptimal provision of options to the patient, in situations where options do indeed exist. In other words, if rational choices are available, the appropriately educated patient should be allowed to "drive the bus." By "driving the bus" I infer active patient participation in the decision-making and strategic treatment-planning process.

The physician must understand that he/she may not have effectively conveyed clinically relevant information to the patient in a form that the patient understands and can digest. The physician should ask the patient to reiterate what they were told to assess the absorption of the critical information. This almost always involves a back-and-forth dialogue between the physician and the patient. A physician monologue, without the assessment of patient information absorption and retention, is a recipe for suboptimal conveyance of critical information. Hence, if gaps in knowledge are identified, the physician should fill them.

If such is accomplished, the patient has "officially" become competent to "drive the bus." The question remains, however, "In what direction?" This is where choices enter the fray. Patients who are given choices become invested in the decision-making process, i.e., they become invested in the driving of the bus in the direction that is best for them, as determined by them. Such choices might include a choice between two medications or the type or extent of surgery to be performed. Regardless of the choices made, the fact that the patient is able to become an integral part of the decision-making team and process (i.e., "driving the bus") increases motivation and compliance.

Physicians should all teach patients to "drive" and allow them to "drive," but with guidance. This, as stated, increases patient compliance. The compliant patient is so much more pleasant and more responsive to treatment than his/her non-compliant counterpart. It all comes down to education and choices.

Section Three

Essay 6
Pseudo-concordance and the Elephant in the Room

Concordance is defined as the presence of agreement or harmony. All of us seek agreement and harmony in most of our daily conversations. Neurosurgeons like to see agreement and harmony—such as between imaging studies and clinical diagnoses. When concordance prevails, we can be relatively confident that our diagnostic accuracy is high. For example, CT evidence of a subdural hematoma (blood clot on the outer surface of the brain) in a patient with a contralateral hemiparesis (opposite-sided weakness) is strongly suggestive of a cause-and-effect relationship between the hematoma and the clinical finding of hemiparesis. The imaging study and the clinical examination are concordant. They are "in agreement," if you will.

Can we be deceived regarding concordance or lack thereof? We sure can. I would like to introduce a term that I find useful—pseudo-concordance. I define pseudo-concordance as: "*An 'apparent' but erroneous relationship between an assumed cause (i.e., imaging study) and an effect (i.e., pain)."* Let me explain by an example. A young male with back pain secondary to undiagnosed ankylosing spondylitis (a disease that stiffens and deforms the spine, beginning in early adulthood) presents with early morning pain that improves with exercise and activity and does not improve with rest (which is characteristic of ankylosing spondylitis). The patient has early morning stiffness that resolves within an hour of awakening. These symptoms are consistent with ankylosing spondylitis (an arthritic condition) related inflammatory pain and are not consistent with mechanical back pain (pain that is deep and agonizing in nature, and that is improved with unloading and worsened by loading the spine) that might be associated with a spondylolisthesis (read on). He, however, presents with an MRI that demonstrates an L4,5 spondylolisthesis (a slippage between the 4th and 5th lumbar vertebrae). The imaging finding (L4,5 spondylolisthesis) is not concordant with the clinical presentation. The patient's symptoms are consistent with ankylosing spondylitis, while the imaging study is consistent with a finding that might cause mechanical back pain,

Section Three

but not the pain endorsed by the patient. However, an unsuspecting physician might make the "erroneous connection" between back pain and the imaging finding (L4,5 spondylolisthesis). The lack of concordance and, in fact, the presence of pseudo-concordance, if missed, could lead to an unnecessary operation (perhaps a spinal fusion) and the overlooking of the diagnosis of ankylosing spondylitis. This places the patient in peril due to the obscuration of the subsequent diagnosis of ankylosing spondylitis by the presence of a failed spine operation and new imaging findings showing screws and rods.

In the this case, the diagnosis of ankylosing spondylosis was overlooked by the physician, who took the imaging finding and clinical finding as concordant when, in fact, they were pseudo-concordant. The physician did not see the "elephant in the room"—i.e., the diagnosis of ankylosing spondylitis. The tragedy here is that the diagnosis of ankylosing spondylitis in this patient may be delayed by years and even decades because the patient had become labeled as a "failed back surgery" patient—thus, overlooking the diagnosis of ankylosing spondylitis. Ankylosing spondylitis related deformity will then gradually progress over time (patients with ankylosing spondylitis often have a progressive kyphosis (bending forward) of the spine).

Now, let's consider a much more common scenario, chronic pain syndrome with back pain and a positive imaging finding, say L4,5 spondylolisthesis. The chronic pain syndrome patient endorses non-restorative sleep and chronic fatigue, is taking opiates for pain, and has pain that is present 24/7. He, however, complains of back pain as his primary complaint. The treating physician could make the erroneous assumption that his pain is related to the imaging finding (L4,5 spondylolisthesis) and, hence, recommend surgery. Such would likely only fuel the fire of the chronic pain syndrome (the patient's true clinical diagnosis) and likely lead to further misery and perhaps further ill-conceived operations and procedures in the future. This represents a pseudo-concordance picture—*"An 'apparent' but erroneous relationship between an assumed cause (i.e., MRI evidence of L4,5 spondylolisthesis) and an effect (i.e., chronic back pain syndrome)."*

In the latter case, the physician, as well, did not see the "elephant in the room"—i.e., the clinical diagnosis of chronic back pain syndrome. How can we learn from this? The simple and effective solution is to establish the clinical diagnosis that is not

Section Three

based on the imaging study, but rather on history and examination. We must distinguish between inflammatory back pain (as seen with ankylosing spondylitis), mechanical back pain, myofascial pain (episodic back muscle spasm-associated pain), and chronic back pain syndrome (as defined above). Each is readily distinguishable from the others. Then, and only then, should the physician look at the imaging study to see if concordance exists. Surgeons and patients alike should be wary of the pitfalls associated with a "pseudo-concordant picture" and make concerted efforts to "see" the elephant in the room. Remember, the elephants are everywhere. The savvy patient may be aware of such misguided decision making. If such is the case, the patient should help right a wrong.

Section Three

Essay 7

"Doctor, I Trust You"

The words "Doctor, I trust you" are possibly the four most meaningful and impactful words uttered by a patient to a physician. They, in essence, convey respect for, and a comfort level with, the physician. In addition, these four words imply that a true and meaningful physician-patient bond has been established.

Trust is earned. It is not given. The keys to earning trust are a sense of competence, honesty, empathy, a genuine expression of caring, affability and listening. Let's start with the sense of competence. I am not sure how one conveys their level of competence. However, to be effective here, the physician must, in fact, be competent. Perhaps an appropriate level of self-confidence on the part of the physician is a good place to start. Humility is critical, so that one does not over- or under-state the level of competence or other physician attributes. Honesty is critical as well. To honestly convey information and answer questions, with an appropriate conveyance of humility, is key.

Empathy and expressing the fact that the physician genuinely cares about the patient engenders a comfort level between the patient and physician that helps seal a bond of trust. Obviously, affability helps. Talking to patients on a human-to-human level engenders trust. It facilitates effective communication, with neither party talking "down" or "up" to the other.

When counseling/informing a patient regarding the risks, benefits, and alternatives of surgery, an honest and comprehensive approach to the discussion is mandatory on the part of the surgeon. The traditional approach to the "informed consent" process should perhaps be re-crafted as an "informed decision-making" process. With the former, the surgeon talks to the patient and informs via a monologue. With the latter, the surgeon and patient interact regarding the risks, benefits and alternatives via a dialogue. They discuss the real risks of surgery, with an emphasis on what really can, but likely will not, go wrong. The patient must take off any blinders that may be

Section Three

present. In other words, the patient and family must carefully consider what all can "go wrong"—not just what they *assume* will "go right."

Perhaps the most important physician attribute here is the art of listening. Physicians learn so much more by listening, —genuinely listening—than by talking. The astute physician will listen and watch for emotions, for hints/clues regarding the establishment of the diagnosis and listen carefully so that the response the physician provides is appropriate and reflective of the fact that he/she *heard* the patient and that he/she cares.

So, if a physician hears from a patient the words "Doctor, I trust you," the physician has scored; but so has the patient. The physician has effectively established an enriched environment that is based on trust. The physician formed a solid team that pits the patient, his/her family, and the physician and his/her team against the enemy—i.e., the disease or pathological process. All are winners here. When this type of enriched environment is established, no matter what happens, the "team" is in it together—win, lose or draw. No lawsuits if things turn out poorly. Just regrets that such happened. On the other hand, if things turn out well, the team can rejoice together as victors and regale themselves with the laurels of victory. Physicians and patients alike, should all strive to achieve these communication goals.

Section Three

Essay 8
Thank You

In the prior essay (Section 3, Essay 7), I discussed the meaningfulness and relevance of the four words "Doctor, I trust you." This trust is earned by the physician and bestowed by the patient. As stated, the keys to earning such trust are a conveyance of competence, honesty, empathy, a genuine expression of caring, affability and listening. The two words "thank you" also are associated with significant meaning and relevance, particularly in the context of the patient-physician relationship. Thank-you's, as opposed to "Doctor, I trust you," go both ways; i.e., from the patient to physician and the physician to patient.

Let us first explore the utterance of a "Thank you" from a patient. In a way, the words "Thank you" convey a similar but less emphatic message to the physician than "Doctor, I trust you." It is an expression of appreciation. Like the words "Doctor, I trust you," physicians should seek to warrant and receive such accolades.

But, what about a "Thank you" utterance from the physician directed to the patient? You might ask, "Why should a physician thank a patient?" Well, first and foremost, without patients physicians would be unemployed. Physicians should be thankful for that alone. More importantly, though, the physician should be thankful for the trust the patient must have had in order to have sought him/her out to be his/her physician. Physicians should also be thankful that the patient felt enough positive karma from the visit to utter the words "Thank you." A return "Thank you" is then most certainly in order, e.g., "Thank you for being you. I truly enjoyed our visit. You have made my day."

Studies have shown that the two words "Thank you," when uttered to the patient by the physician, are associated with greater patient satisfaction. If a patient hears the words "Thank you" from a physician, he/she should feel that, in a way, a communication victory was achieved.

So, to the physician, do not hesitate to thank the patient, and make it genuine. Say it often. This, in turn, translates into gratitude and an increased satisfaction with

Section Three

care. This, then, translates into improved physician satisfaction. To the patient, the words "Thank you" mean more than the physician may think. It is the little things that enrich lives via fulfillment and positive karma. It is the little things that cause the physician, at the end of a day, to think, *Today was a good day.* ☺

Section Three

Essay 9

"I'm Sorry"

The words "I'm sorry" are commonly uttered. The true meaning of "I'm sorry," however, varies, depending on context. If a surgeon's patient experiences an adverse surgical outcome, the words "I'm sorry" are often associated with much more complex considerations than the words "I'm sorry" itself conveys. For example, the context is in striking contrast to a situation that is associated with the expression of concern to an individual who just stubbed his toe and is in pain, or even the expression of concern to a friend who recently lost a loved one.

In the case of an adverse outcome, the surgeon must be careful to differentiate between being sorry that the adverse outcome occurred, i.e., being sorry for the outcome (implying that bad things happen, and all were aware that such could be the outcome of surgery) versus being sorry that the surgeon caused the adverse outcome (implying the admission of responsibility and/or guilt).

Most but not all adverse outcomes are not the result of a mistake, but rather the result of one or both of two circumstances that are often outside the control of the surgeon. Some may be the result of a decision that, in retrospect, was a decision that led to an unanticipated suboptimal outcome. "In retrospect," or the use of the proverbial "retro-spect-a-scope," implies that one could not predict the outcome of any given approach in advance, but the clarity of the "suboptimal choice" appears obvious after the outcome is realized. Such outcomes are the result of a judgment call. Most judgment calls are made when two or more choices are in consideration for the determination of a strategic decision. Often, multiple alternatives are reasonable. The choice of one of the reasonable alternatives, however, may lead down the pathway to an adverse outcome. The alternatives should be discussed preoperatively when the discussion leads to the consideration of "risks, benefits and alternatives." The term equipoise is relevant here. Clinical equipoise, in the modern-day medical vernacular, is a term that is used to describe the extent of uncertainty regarding the determination of the best

Section Three

approach to a clinical problem (equipoise is discussed in greater detail in Section 3, Essay 12). When there is significant disagreement amongst experts regarding the best approach to a problem, significant equipoise exists.

The second type of adverse outcome that is outside the control of the surgeon is the result of what some term an "act of God" ("act of God" is a common term used to define circumstances that are beyond one's control). Unanticipated hemorrhage and excessive blood loss or unanticipated difficulties with tumor dissection are examples of such "acts of God" that can convert a smooth, uneventful operation into a catastrophe.

It should be obvious that being "sorry" that an adverse outcome occurred is in stark contrast to being "sorry" that the surgeon him/herself caused the adverse outcome. The surgeon must differentiate between the two in his/her mind and then convey the appropriate message to the patient and family. The conveyance of "being sorry" that an adverse outcome occurred, rather than "being sorry" that the surgeon caused the adverse outcome, is perhaps more effectively accomplished via non-verbal communication than with verbal communication. Empathy and the art of expressing the fact that one cares tends to cause the patient and family to trust the surgeon. Trust is the key here. "Doc, we know that you did your best." The surgeon must, however, genuinely have earned the trust and must be "sorry" for the right reason.

Empathic communication begins long before the incision is made. Informed decision making (the broader context within which informed consent is taken) that is based on facts, trust, and the honest portrayal of the risks, benefits and alternatives associated with the surgical intervention is a critical component of the process. It is emphasized that the preoperative establishment of mutual trust between the patient and family and the surgeon establishes a solid foundation for any and all postoperative discussions. Based on such a foundation, the words "I'm sorry" become an empathic utterance, which may need little or no explanation. Subsequent conversations, with the liberal expression of empathy, often help all involved parties through this difficult time. Again, mutual trust is the key. Such is difficult to establish after the adverse event has occurred if mutual trust was not established before.

Finally, if the surgeon caused the adverse outcome via a mistake or error, the words "I'm sorry" remain appropriate, but must be stated within the context of a very

Section Three

different set of circumstances. First and foremost, such conversations are clearly facilitated by the surgeon having already established a preoperative high level of trust and a bond with the patient and family. In this situation, the surgeon should take responsibility for the adverse outcome. In many institutions, it is appropriate to do such with legal guidance. Regardless, honesty is clearly the best policy. Attempts at a cover-up rarely succeed and are clearly disingenuous and dishonest. Empathetically expressing concern and regret can be cathartic for the surgeon and begin the emotional healing process for the patient and family, as well as the surgeon.

Bad outcomes happen. Neurosurgeons see them more than most medical specialists. Dealing with bad outcomes should be part of a surgeon's communication repertoire, with the establishment of appropriate and strong lines of communication with patients and their families. Both the physician and the patient must strive to create an environment of trust that is based on honesty. This is facilitated by the establishment of a bond that connects the surgeon with the patient and family. Empathy! Empathy! Empathy!

Section Three

Essay 10
The Breakpoint

"The lesson seems almost Zen: you live longer only when you stop trying to live longer."
– Atul Gawande from *Being Mortal: Medicine and What Matters in the End*

Breakpoint (definition: a place or time at which an interruption or change is made) is a term that not uncommonly is used to define a transition from one way or strategy to another. Atul Gawande, in his book *Being Mortal: Medicine and What Matters in the End*, dwells on and elaborates upon the importance of the breakpoint regarding the care of patients with terminal diseases, such as cancer. In such cases, the breakpoint is that point in the care of the patient where the strategic plan is altered from one of "fighting" for increasing length of life (time) to quality of life (e.g., quality time with family and being home rather than in the hospital)—the scenes, the odors, the loved ones, the calm, the peace, the once small things in life that have become oh so much more important as the end draws near.

Indeed, Gawande's statement "The lesson seems almost Zen: you live longer only when you stop trying to live longer" is, in fact, based on prior published research that is outlined in his book. Physicians seemingly perpetually focus on length of life. They quote statistics, complication rates with surgery, and various other factors to fashion a projection regarding length of life. They often discuss these variables and projections with the patient and family. However, do they always give the patient the knowledge base to make rational decisions regarding what remains of their life? The patient, the family and treating physicians often get sucked into a vortex of decision making that considers predominantly length of life, e.g., life expectancy without surgery six months vs. nine months with surgery. However, even with a good surgical outcome, some of the hypothetical extra three months of life is spent in postoperative pain and discomfort—and what if complications ensue? Duration of life may have been extended, but at what quality of life-related cost?

Section Three

As I think of prior experiences with terminal patients, my mind keeps bringing me back to a 40ish-year-old patient and father of several young teenagers and a loving wife. He had a metastatic cancer involving his skull base with erosion of his occipital condyle (the platform that connects the skull to the upper cervical spine) unilaterally with lower brain and nerve dysfunction that resulted in difficult swallowing, and aspiration (inability to prevent saliva and food from going into the airways and lungs). He had significant head and neck pain. The patient, his wife, and referring physicians applied immense pressures on me to perform an occiput-cervical stabilization operation (screws and rods that would rigidly connect the skull to the upper cervical spine and, thus, stabilize the affected area) for pain. My assessment of this situation unveiled the following: 1) His life expectancy appeared to be in the range of one to five months; 2) his pain was predominantly nocturnal (maximum in evening), and not so much mechanical (pain due to abnormal motion where the tumor eroded bone) in nature; and 3) he was miserable in the hospital and in his hospital bed. What does a life expectancy of one to five months mean in the big scheme of things? Should we strive for five months? Why? His pain was nocturnal and, by the way, not related to motion (mechanical). This suggests a biologic pain component (low nocturnal cortisol levels leading to increased pain when the sun sets). It was not surprising that he was miserable in the hospital—the sterile and foreign environment that it is.

So, we instituted evening low-dose steroid administration to treat his low cortisol levels. We provided a collar for comfort. He responded with diminished pain. He was discharged to home to sleep with his wife and be with his children. He touched them, was comforted by them and loved by them—in his own home!

He died at home under hospice care (consultation) in three months. We did not operate. We did not inflict more pain. We did embrace the breakpoint. We collectively quit being concerned about length of life. We collectively began to emphasize the importance of quality of life and strove to optimize such. In the end, he died in his own bed at home—with his family, all comfortable with their choices and the inevitable end result.

This case was transformative for me. I truly saw, and was able to embrace, the meaning of the "breakpoint." Neurosurgeons have difficulty with "watching a patient

Section Three

die" while not doing something to help. The point here, though, is that the neurosurgeon is not "watching the patient die," he/she is "allowing the patient to live" the highest-quality life possible in the time that remains. Perhaps surgeons should set, with the patient and family of a terminal patient, a breakpoint—beyond which we seek only to optimize quality of life and essentially ignore longevity. After all, when we do such it appears that patients live longer as well. "The lesson seems almost Zen: you live longer only when you stop trying to live longer."

Section Three

Essay 11
Dogma, Cost, and Healthcare

"That's one small step for man, one giant leap for mankind."
– Neil Armstrong

"It ain't what you don't know that gets you into trouble.
It's what you know for sure that just ain't so." – Mark Twain (Sachel Paige)

An article by Kumar et al, published in *World Neurosurgery* [1], presented compelling evidence to suggest that neurosurgeons traditionally have over-imaged (with CT) mild head injury patients with subarachnoid hemorrhage (blood in the spinal fluid spaces that surround the brain. The article demonstrated no ill effect associated with eliminating repeat CT in neurologically stable patients.

On the surface, one might think, *So what! Yes, we can diminish the use of unnecessary imaging studies and diminish radiation exposure, but such is but a "nano-scopic" element of the overall health care costs and safety considerations.* But, is it?

Ecker et al [2], in his accompanying invited Perspective on the Kumar et al paper, emphasized the quadruple aim of health-care decision making and resourcing: 1. enhancing patient experience, 2. improving population health, 3. reducing costs, and 4. improving the life of healthcare workers. He suggested that the Kumar et al paper focused directly on the quadruple aim. In a broader scheme, such a focus could not only could lead to a safer environment for patients and caregivers, but also save hundreds of millions of dollars in the process.

Ecker et al emphasized that "Rules and regulations that present a safety risk for patients must be challenged. Entrenched dogmas and fear of medicolegal repercussions need to be replaced by objective clinical research translated into practice." Ecker suggests that we must aggressively challenge inappropriate dogma and strive to diminish cost in a safe, patient and provider centric manner.

Section Three

James Van Dellen [3], in his similarly invited Perspective to the Kumar et al paper, eloquently states, "Challenging prevailing views at all levels and thereby developing new concepts in Medicine is not only innovative but the essential core in our progress to improve our care and to meet our responsibilities to our patients."

Via multiple small steps (akin to the small step of Neil Armstrong), we can make huge changes. We can only accomplish such, though, by remaining poised to challenge dogma—and, in turn, being receptive to being challenged. Van Dellen refers to such as aligning with the Socratic principles of questioning and challenging. He suggests that we should adhere to these principles that are associated with challenging convention and the acceptance of being challenged.

Mark Twain, and later Sachel Paige, alluded to an arrogance that, to one degree or another, we all harbor: "It ain't what you don't know that gets you into trouble. It's what you know for sure that just ain't so." Van Dellen refers to this arrogance as well. He states that "Dogma and unchallenged arrogance in 'knowledge' leads to stagnant thought and stultified progression, and persistence of managements which may be of no benefit to a patient. It may, however, elevate the standing of the practitioner, both pecuniary and socially." Self-interests, including financial, academic and other self-interests, can lead to biases that ultimately result in suboptimal care and increased cost. No one wins here, except for the guilty perpetrators of bias. The acceptance of randomized control trials as "gospel," for example, can be dangerous from a quality and cost of healthcare perspective (remember the reference to Mark Twain and Satchel Paige). We all must appropriately challenge dogmas. We must strive to achieve excellence. Unfortunately, it is far easier, though, to accept than it is to challenge.

Van Dellen refers to an analogy by comparing the "Art of Medicine" and the "Science of Medicine." We tend to look for "evidence"—i.e., evidence-based medicine ("Science of Medicine"). We evidently do not accept the fact that to some degree the literature is flawed. It is through the application of the "Art of Medicine" that we see gaps and flaws in our knowledge base and then begin to challenge dogmas. Van Dellen states, in this regard, that "the 'Art of Medicine' is becoming overwhelmed by the rigid structures of the 'Science of Medicine,' by which it is believed can be practiced purely quantitatively and not with the importance of more variable and sensible qualitative input."

Section Three

With our current and increasing focus on data that is derived from the "Science of Medicine," physicians have tended to disregard individual thought and, in a sense, became less patient centric. Physicians can resist this dangerous trend. They can challenge dogma, as have Kumar et al. Goren et al, [4] in a third invited Perspective, states: "This article (the article by Kumar et al regarding over imaging) should serve as the beginning of a conversation about the most appropriate and efficient use of our healthcare resources." Let us look for more dogmas to "bust." Physicians should embrace the "Art of Medicine" and begin to challenge the "Science of Medicine." In so doing, we can possibly make the medical world a better place.

Endnotes

1. Kumar A, Alvarado A, Shah K, Arnold PM. Necessity of repeat CT imaging in isolated mild traumatic subarachnoid hemorrhage. World Neurosurg. 2018;113:399-403.
2. Ecker, RD. NoNeed for Repeat Imaging in Patients with Mild Traumatic Subarachnoid Hemorrhage without Clinical Progression. World Neurosurg. 2018;113:404-405.
3. van Dellen JR. Big Little Challenges. World Neurosurg. 2018;113:406-408.
4. Goren O, Griessenauer CJ, Schirmer CM. Do We Really Need to Repeat Computed Tomography Imaging in Isolated Mild Traumatic Subarachnoid Hemorrhage? World Neurosurg. 2018;113:409-410.

Section Three

Essay 12
Clinical Equipoise

> Equipoise: "1: a state of equilibrium. 2: counterbalance."
> – Merriam Webster

In the medical arena, the use of the term equipoise has been steadily increasing over the past decade. The Merriam Webster definition of equipoise does not adequately reflect the use of the term in the clinical and research arenas. In these clinically oriented venues, the term equipoise refers to situations in which there is uncertainty or conflicting expert opinion regarding diagnostic, prevention, or treatment options. Equipoise in medicine, in a sense, is a measure of uncertainty regarding the most appropriate treatment, diagnostic or prevention strategy choice. Situations in which significant equipoise exists lend themselves to research to determine the truth or best way to manage a patient or a population of patients. Such research, if done properly (i.e., seeking to find the truth via exploratory inquiry and not to prove a point via conclusion-based research), narrows the uncertainty/equipoise gap in knowledge.

"Clinical equipoise is the assumption that there is not one 'better' intervention present (for either the control or experimental group) during the design of a randomized controlled trial (RCT). A true state of equipoise exists when for a choice between two or more care options."[1] In such cases, clinicians must make a decision regarding their own best judgment, which is based on the experience of the clinician, as well as his/her assessment of the literature. Clinician bias inevitably plays a role in the decision-making process. After all, it is abundantly clear to most clinicians that there is "more than one way to skin a cat" (in this circumstance, a colloquialism that implies that there exist multiple treatment modalities that may be used to achieve success in any given clinical situation). The recent randomized trial regarding the management of cervical spondylotic myelopathy, published in *JAMA,* is a great example. Three treatment options for cervical spondylotic myelopathy were studied: anterior decompression and fusion, posterior la-

Section Three

minectomy and fusion, and laminoplasty.[2] All three treatment modalities effectively managed myelopathy and no clear differences in outcome between the three groups were identified. So, what is a surgeon to do when confronted with a clinical treatment dilemma, with which there is significant equipoise regarding management? The surgeon must use his/her best judgment and rely on an assessment of the literature. In other words, the surgeon should/must do what works best in his/her hands.

We must study high equipoise "situations/scenarios" in order to narrow the knowledge gap regarding treatment and diminish the overall burden of equipoise. Non-biased randomized clinical trials are a means of diminishing the burden of equipoise. "The concept of 'equipoise,' or the 'uncertainty principle,' has been represented as a central ethical principle, and holds that a subject may be enrolled in a randomized controlled trial (RCT) only if there is true uncertainty about which of the trial arms is most likely to benefit the patient."[3] The term "non-biased trial" is the operative phrase here. We know that many randomized trials have subsequently been shown to be flawed.[4] Such research is most often conclusion-based research that was performed with the intent of proving a point, rather than seeking the truth; hence significant bias is introduced into study design, patient selection, and outcome assessment. We must strive to seek the truth and to cast our biases aside. In the words of Mark Twain: "It ain't what you don't know that gets you into trouble. It's what you know for sure that just ain't so." So, cast biases aside and seek to determine the truth. Only then can we effectively reduce the burden of equipoise. In many ways, the discussion pertains to life in general. We should always seek the truth and limit bias in the research and decision-making arenas.

Endnotes

1. Cook, C. Clinical equipoise and personal equipoise: two necessary ingredients for reducing bias in manual therapy trials. *J Man Manip Ther.* 2011 Feb.; 19(1): 55–57. doi: *10.1179/106698111X12899036752014.*
2. Ghogawala, Z.; et al. Effect of Ventral vs. Dorsal Spinal Surgery on Patient-Reported Physical Functioning in Patients with Cervical Spondylotic Myelopathy: A Randomized Clinical Trial. *JAMA.* 2021; 325(10): 942-951. Doi:10.1001/jama.2021.1233.

Section Three

3. Fries, J. F.; and E. Krishnan. Equipoise, design bias, and randomized controlled trials: the elusive ethics of new drug development. *Arthritis Res Ther.* 2004; 6(3): R250–R255. Published online: 2004 Mar. 18. Doi: *10.1186/ar1170*.
4. Lehrer, J. The Truth Wears Off—Is There Something Wrong with the Scientific Method? Annals of Science, December 13, 2010.

Section Three

Essay 13
Fulfillment and Meaning

"The most important human endeavor is the striving for morality in our actions. Our inner balance and even our existence depend on it. Only morality in our actions can give beauty and dignity to life. To make this a living force and bring it to clear consciousness is perhaps the foremost task of education."

– Albert Einstein

Albert Einstein was a secular humanist and a supporter of the Ethical Culture Movement. He believed that "a man's ethical behavior should be based on sympathy, education and social ties." He feared that the discoveries he made might be exploited with evil intent, which perhaps is why he emphasizes the point that "only morality in our actions can give beauty and dignity to life." Regardless, the quote by Einstein is exemplary of his quest for fulfillment and meaning.

I am going to take the bold liberty here of adding one word to the end of his quote for the purposes of discussion. The word is "communication." It is via communication that we express our fears, our thoughts, our opinions and our love or disdain for others. It is how we express sympathy, how we educate and the mechanism by which we relate to others. Perhaps, most importantly, communication is our conduit to all others.

It is through education and communication that we achieve fulfillment and meaning. Conversely and sadly, it may also be the way we create stress and unhappiness. Effective communication with others almost universally involves empathy and sympathy. Empathic (expressing the fact that one cares) and sympathetic (an understanding and appreciation of another's woes) communication is self-fulfilling and, hence, "gives beauty and dignity to life."

Of course, we strive to perform our duties well. The achievement of good results for a surgeon demands that he/she does far more than a well-executed operation. It

Section Three

involves a consideration of the *how, the what and the why*. A well-executed operation entails the provision of meticulous attention to detail regarding the intricacy and complexity of an operation done well, i.e., the *how*. The *what and why*, however, play an equally if not more important role. The well-executed operation is only a part of *how* a surgeon achieves surgical success. Success also depends on choosing the right operation (the *what*) and the decision to operate in the first place (the *why*). A well-executed operation is for naught if it does not match the patient's clinical needs. A painstaking approach to the mechanics of the surgical decision-making process is clearly warranted. It is, indeed, fulfilling for the surgeon to have performed a well-executed operation that involves the consideration of the *how, the what and the why*. Perhaps what is most fulfilling, though, is what happens before and after the operation and, in the case of a non-operative patient, what transpires as the physician informs the patient and family and helps them make often difficult and critical decisions.

Empathically helping patients through the operative decision-making process, and postoperative trials and tribulations provide meaning to physicians and surgeons—at least it should. Empathically helping terminal patients strategically wander through the abyss of difficult decisions, for which they are initially ill equipped to make, is indeed fulfilling. Becoming a "beacon" who helps guide the patient and family through the aforementioned abyss creates a bond that should be, in and of itself, the physician's ultimate reward. It is, in this way, that "doing what's right" becomes the surgeon's own personal beacon that guides the surgeon to a fulfilled and meaningful life.

Physicians must perpetually ask themselves the following questions: How can I empathically lead others to a better place? How can I most effectively serve others? Am I effectively expressing the fact that I care? How can I become an even better leader than I currently am? How can I make the next version of me better than the current one? These questions involve, at their core, effective communication. It is through this relentless pursuit of self-improvement that physicians truly achieve fulfillment and meaning in life. Patients and caregivers alike benefit.

Section Three

Essay 14
Highs and Lows

Why is it that a sports team at any level can win against seemingly insurmountable odds and then lose to a much lesser opponent in the next game? The high after an unlikely victory is expected. Jubilant is the victor. So, why does the next game so often result in diametrically opposite results—i.e., defeat? Some say, and rightfully so, that complacency follows a jubilant victory. Complacency, is that the reason for the unpredictable loss? Maybe! Maybe not!

Good coaches understand this and continuously emphasize the importance of minimizing the peak of the highs and, conversely, the "valley" associated with the lows. Maintaining an emotional even keel between the highs and lows would seem to be prudent in sports.

But doesn't this phenomenon apply to non-sports activities and to life in general? From the perspective of a neurosurgeon, "snatching a patient from the jaws of death" with a technically difficult and well-done operation is deserving of a little self-adulation, but just a little—and then move on. The neurosurgeon should not be so full of him or herself that the "high" associated with the "victory" permeates into the realms of further thoughts and decisions. One should never derive the conclusion that "I now have no limits." The ability of the neurosurgeon to effectively negotiate the emotional abyss of incredible successes with only a modicum of self-adulation may prepare him/her for the inevitable failure or complication. It might even diminish complication rates if the surgeon maintains a realistic "handle" on his/her true capabilities—thus, not coming away from a "high" with the notion that "I can fix anything!!!!!"

Neurosurgeons, in general, tend to let themselves experience high highs and very low lows. I have become increasingly aware of this as I age. I tolerate complications much less effectively than I did twenty years prior. I dwell on them. I can't get them out of my mind. It takes a long time for me to begin to emotionally recover from a complication. That's not good. Do I overreact to the highs, thus causing me to dwell

Section Three

on the lows? I don't think so, but it's possible. I don't think that I have big swings of jubilance—but am I fooling myself? Are these swings escalating as I age? I cannot answer these questions. I can only speculate that I should attempt to modulate the "mood swings." As they say, "everything in moderation."

Isn't life like this in general, though? We all should modulate the highs and lows for our own sanity and self-preservation. Unfortunately, most of us fall short of such. Sports teams continue to falter in the game following a miraculous victory—even in the presence of great coaching. It all comes down to the intangible emotions, feelings, and triggers that, in turn, affect our performance as individuals and as teams. If someone has this figured out, let me know so that we can share it with the world.

Section Three

Essay 15

What the Pandemic Has Taught Us

The good derived from the COVID-19 pandemic pales in comparison with the bad. However, the COVID-19 pandemic has taught many of us to be cognizant of kindness and to exhibit greater patience. It also has arguably caused some of us to live with situations that are out of our control. This represents the glass-half-full mentality. I would add to this list of positives, the rapid development and deployment of virtual communication platforms that have revolutionized local, regional, national and international education and communication, as well as medical advances, such as vaccines and advanced therapeutic strategies.

However, the glass-half-empty posture has led many to emphasize the overwhelmingly negative aspect of the pandemic. Let us begin with the loss of thousands of lives, disruption of lifestyle, loss of jobs and isolationism related depression and related mood disorders.

Also, a poorly veiled downside of the pandemic has been the discourse and disharmony associated with mask wearing, vaccinations, and social distancing. It is a sad day when politics trump science and the recommendations of medical scholars and scientists are criticized by those who have no prior or acquired knowledge in the medical and related scientific fields.

To put the collateral benefits of the pandemic into perspective, both the good and bad sequelae of the pandemic must be considered. Perhaps, then, we will be able to more clearly "see" the perspective regarding collateral benefits.

Without question, the loss of lives and the pandemic-related financial devastation have been crippling. Regardless, let us take this aspect of the pandemic off the table for the remainder of this discussion. With this obvious negative component off the table, our consideration then focuses on the collateral benefits and negatives.

Obviously, we as a community of humans living on planet earth have become, to a large extent, more cognizant of kindness and for the most part become more patient

Section Three

and tolerant. We, indeed, have learned to live with situations that are out of our control. Perhaps, most importantly, we humans rapidly developed and deployed virtual communication platforms and have, through innovation and collaboration, developed lifesaving tests, drugs, and clinical strategies to fight the demonic COVID-19 virus.

In the previous paragraph I used phrases such as "to a large extent" and "for the most part." This is to emphasize that not all of us have become more cognizant of kindness, nor have all of us become more patient, etc. The disruption of lifestyle, loss of jobs, isolationism, and ensuing discourse that is often vitriolic and at times hostile have been prevalent and, occasionally, have surpassed the "boiling point."

Hostility and the vitriolic discord have divided us and have unquestionably been obstructive of political progress, while playing a role in the less-than-optimal management of the pandemic from a public health and medical perspective. Arguably, politics have indeed trumped science during these trying times.

In the end, we all need to come together to solve problems, without conflict escalation. Rather than succumbing to the latter, we must seek conflict resolution. This will not be easy. There are a lot of wounds to heal. They can only be healed by communication and compromise.

We, however, should also rejoice in our triumphs. For those of us who have become more tolerant, kind and patient—keep it going. Such can be contagious. For those of us who have succumbed to the vitriol and discord, seek resolution via communication and compromise. Then and only then can we begin to heal.

Let us all step back, take a deep breath, hold, and then exhale—as we think these words: "I can do this by doing my part."

Section Three

Essay 16

Defining Limits

What makes neurosurgeons tick? What drives them? First of all, nearly all surgeons, to one degree or another, are thrill seekers. They "live" for the thrill of affecting change in the course of their patients' lives via quick and decisive action. In a way, surgeons performing high risk surgery are seeking "thrill." They, however, often have other non-clinical "drivers of thrill." For me, it is running. I have run since high school and oftentimes, what I now realize, I have run excessively (an estimated 70,000 – 80,000 miles in my lifetime). I have run over fifty marathons, multiple quarter- and half-triathlons, two full-length triathlons, and an additional annual "self-challenge" event that, if you will, ultimately 'uncovered' a limit.

From age 40 to age 64, I ran my age in miles in one setting annually, in some approximation to my birthday. At age 40, it was a "piece of cake." At age 64 I, however, reached my limit. As each year passed, I naturally became slower due to natural senescence. It, hence, took longer for me to train for the event, as the event became more arduous (by one additional mile) each year. In a way, the converging limitations associated with the ever-increasing time required to train and the degree of difficulty associated with the run itself caused me to end my "self-challenge." I reached and defined my limit.

My story does not end here, though. I became slower and slower—nothing like the "fleet of foot" guy I used to be. I developed symptomatic atrial fibrillation which, at least in part, is related to the excessive exercise strategy that I partook in and enjoyed. I failed medical therapy and two cardioversions. I then had a successful cardiac ablation. I am now on a blood thinner. All of this for running. I would do it again, though. I defined a limit that tested my "metal"—not unlike taking on difficult and risky surgical procedures. Both have made and currently help make me stronger.

I now slowly run twenty miles a week in four five-mile segments. This is a far cry from fifty or more miles per week. I now run for the health of it and not to excess. I

Section Three

run to be with my dog, Blue, in the forest. I lament the pace at which I run and the cardiac issues I have, but I still run. My wife Mary astutely often says, *"Running, in part, defines who you (me) are."* She also states to me, *"I don't know what you (me) would do if you could not run."* I think she is right. Running is a part of my persona, along with so many other activities, including being a neurosurgeon.

I ran and defined a physical limit. I care for patients and continue to "enjoy" the stresses and thrill associated with tough and risky operations—with the significant rewards associated with success. Reaching one's limit (defining a limit) makes one stronger. Running, I truly believe, makes me a better surgeon.

Defining limits seems so simple, but it's not. It took me a better part of a lifetime to truly define a physical limit. I am not different from most others. Most people set and define limits. Understanding the extent to which we can push ourselves helps us understand ourselves. My advice, determine what drives you and define your limits.

Section Three

Essay 17
Less Can Be More

"I didn't have time to write a short letter, so I wrote a long one instead."
— Mark Twain

"I have made this longer than usual, because I have not had time to make it shorter."
— Blaise Pascal

Recently, one of **WORLD NEUROSURGERY**'s esteemed board members and section editor, Russell Andrews, pointed out an interesting article from the April 17, 2021, issue of *The Economist*.[1] In this article, the notion that, to improve something, *"adding new things rather than stripping back what is already there, even when additions lead to sub-par results"* is a common error. They point out that humans struggle with "subtractive thinking." When asked to improve by modification, most humans (roughly 80%) will add something rather than subtract a component (roughly 20%).

The two quotes by Mark Twain and Blaise Pascal refer to the same phenomenon as it is associated with writing. From a medical journal editor's perspective, one of the most common errors associated with submitted manuscripts is the lack of brevity—in other words, the manuscript is far too verbose: *"I have not had time to make it shorter."*

Over seven years ago, we at **WORLD NEUROSURGERY** initiated a section termed "Doing More with Less." Over the years, **WORLD NEUROSURGERY** has published many articles in this section, addressing creative solutions to clinical problems in resource-challenged environments. Not only did the many published solutions solve problems with fewer resources; oftentimes the solution was the best solution regardless of the extent of access to resources.

Leidy Klotz opined on this subject, *"Subtraction is the act of getting to less, but it is not the same as doing less. In fact, getting to less often means doing, or at least thinking,*

Section Three

more."[2] This is precisely what Twain and Pascal were referring to, as it pertains to writing, with their quotes.

Neurosurgeons, as well as most physicians, and most people for that matter, are enamored by technologies that we think makes us more efficient and better at what we do. Technologies, however, do not make us better surgeons or better engineers, teachers, or attorneys. In fact, many new technologies often cause us to do less, think less and perhaps become less proficient. The technology replaces the doing, thinking, and the honing of skills that make us what we strive for—competence, proficiency, forward thinking, etc. This can be a slippery slope. We must aggressively avoid becoming enamored with and subservient to technology.

Technological advances, in addition, can lead surgeons and others to do more, often more than they should. Often, because of a technology related false sense of security, a less skillful surgeon becomes self-empowered to do more surgery—and as implied above, perhaps too much surgery. A false sense of confidence can be, indeed, dangerous. This is a component of the Dunning-Kruger Effect, discussed in Section 2, Essay 18.

For a surgeon to be skilled and able to perform at a high level is imperative. As alluded to herein, new technologies can cause the surgeon to use the technologies as a replacement for the development and maturation of his/her surgical acumen. This can be dangerous. Such can enable surgeons with substandard skillsets to perform operations, without a solid clinical acumen and skillset foundation. Conversely, new technologies can help make a good or great surgeon even better. Hence the thoughtful and measured utilization of technologies by competent and skillful surgeons should be the norm. This applies to people in all walks of life.

The mark of a good surgeon is the ability to achieve good outcomes by utilizing available resources. This good surgeon may, indeed, often find that less is more. Perhaps "subtractive thinking" should become a part of our vernacular for all of us – not just surgeons.

Section Three

Endnotes

1. Why People Forget That Less Is Often More. The Economist, April 17, 2021. (*https://www.economist.com/science-and-technology/2021/04/14/why-people-forget-that-less-is-often-more*).

2. Klotz, L. Subtract: Why Getting to Less Can Mean Thinking More. *www.behavioralscientist.org*. May 12, 2021 (*https://behavioralscientist.org/subtract-why-getting-to-less-can-mean-thinking-more/*).

Section Three

Essay 18
The Good Old Days

> *"We can never know about the days to come*
> *But we think about them anyway*
> *And I wonder if I'm really with you now*
> *Or just chasin' after some finer day*
> *… And tomorrow we might not be together*
> *I'm no prophet and I don't know nature's ways*
> *So I'll try and see into your eyes right now*
> *And stay right here 'cause these are the good old days…"*
> – Carly Simon (American songwriter and singer. Lyrics taken from the 1971 hit song "Anticipation.")

> *"It was the best of times, it was the worst of times…."*
> – Charles Dickens (excerpt from *Tale of Two Cities*)

> *"I want war. To me all means will be right. My motto is not 'Don't, whatever you do, annoy the enemy.' My motto is 'Destroy him by all and any means.'"*
> – Adolf Hitler

Ah, yes, the good old days. Weren't they wonderful? We yearn for them. In the "before," that time prior to early 2020 beginning of the COVID-19 pandemic, we were functioning as usual. Well, maybe not so much. There was significant political and racial strife worldwide. Regardless, I ask the question, were *"the good old days"* really that good?

We humans yearn for our memories of days gone by. The operative word here though, is "memories." Our memories tend to be selective. We tend to remember good things that happened to us and block out the bad. With so much strife and so

Section Three

many natural disasters, including war and climate change related catastrophes, it is difficult to think that *"these are the good old days…,"* as opined by Carly Simon. I will, hence, dwell on the notion that we may, indeed, be amidst *"the good old days"* as we look to the future.

History repeats itself. There have always been tyrants and cruel people, I would guess, since the dawn of mankind. Human beings have been victimized via acts of cruelty and genocide at the hands of tyrants. From these episodes of tyranny, though, some good emerges and then flourishes. Charles Dickens opens his novel *A Tale of Two Cities* with *"It was the best of times, it was the worst of times, it was the age of wisdom, it was the age of foolishness, it was the epoch of belief, it was the epoch of incredulity.…"* This describes where we sit right now in the middle of a pandemic, climate change, racial unrest, the Putin war, etc.. We fear the worst, such as Putin taking on the persona of Hitler, particularly as we take note of Hitler's quote: *"I want war. To me all means will be right. My motto is not 'Don't, whatever you do, annoy the enemy.' My motto is 'Destroy him by all and any means.'"* Interestingly, NATO's, the United States' and many other nation's philosophy is to not annoy Putin. He apparently does not care about lives lost and human suffering. Yes, he, indeed, could be pushed to initiate a nuclear war.

How then can this be "the best of times" or *"the good old days"*? Hope springs eternal. As a result of all the converging catastrophes, many nations have begun working in unison, we have a renewed focus on civil rights, a more unified attack on global warming, etc. We humans are resilient. We do not advance by lamenting *"the good old days."* Down the road, we indeed may look back at today and say, "Those were the good old days." To help ensure that this happens, we must all work together to overcome obstacles and right the existing wrongs, hopefully via diplomacy and the advancement of technology, science, and medicine.

Let us make these days *"the good old days."* Let us all collaborate with a purpose. Let us not seek strife. Let us strive to make these days "the good days" of tomorrow.

Section Three

Essay 19
Comparison is the Thief of Joy

"Comparison is the thief of joy."
– Theodore Roosevelt, 26th President of the United States

"Dunning-Kruger Effect: A hypothetical cognitive bias stating that people with low ability at a task overestimate their own ability and people with high ability at a task underestimate their own ability."
– Definition from Wikipedia, paraphrased

Yes, indeed, *"comparison is the thief of joy."* When we compare ourselves to others or what we have versus what others have, we generally become jealous and feel inferior or jubilant and boastful. Not much good comes from such comparisons. According to Amy Silver[1], *"the process of constantly evaluating our own behavior, thoughts, emotions, relationships, jobs, houses, clothes, looks, lives to each other is one of the most damaging internal narratives we can have. It can make us miserable as we assess our own situations in comparison to the world of others."* Of significant note from a historical perspective, there are a number of biblical references admonishing the comparison of oneself to others.

If such comparisons are so harmful, why do we make them? Perhaps, in some cases, comparisons provide a façade of superiority, behind which we can hide. If I believe that I am a better doctor, engineer, mom, or runner than the comparator, one could create a protective shell that can dangerously cause one to develop and nurture an elitist attitude—an attitude that is perceived by others as "being full of yourself."

At the opposite pole, feelings of inferiority may emerge, as the affected individual becomes jealous for not being as fast, as smart, as wealthy as the comparator. This discussion is interestingly and almost eerily parallel to the discussion regarding the Dunning-Kruger Effect, documented in Section 2 Essay 18 as *"a hypothetical cognitive bias stating that people with low ability at a task overestimate their own ability and people*

Section Three

with high ability at a task underestimate their own ability." The revelation for me here is that the "comparison" of oneself with others initiates the polarized response associated with the Dunning-Kruger Effect. Those with a high level of ability underestimate their own ability, thus resulting in an inferiority complex of sorts. This has been termed "The Imposter Syndrome," the topic of Section 2, essay 16 herein. Conversely, those with low ability tend to overestimate their own ability.

Again, nothing good comes from such comparisons with others. Perhaps what we should do is strive to be competent and not let internally contrived comparison with others get in the way of our goal: competence.

So, how do we liberate ourselves from this "comparison quagmire"? It's simple: Do not compare ourselves to others. More easily said than done. Amy Silver, in the previously referenced article herein, has five recommendations, each of which she clarifies and elaborates upon: 1. Recognize when you are most susceptible to comparison; 2. Practice self-compassion; 3. Consider other perspectives; 4. Take action; and 5. Don't let fear paralyze you. For further clarification, I encourage you to read her article.[1]

My take on this: Try to simply avoid comparison with others. It is not healthy. Try to maintain an equilibrium—that is an equilibrium between over- and under-estimating our abilities. Do not get too full of ourselves. I struggle with these things. I am sure most of us do. Acquiring an understanding of the issues involved and honesty assessing ourself is key.

Comparison is, indeed, the thief of joy. We all must strive to liberate ourselves from comparisons with others, particularly those comparisons that threaten our wellbeing.

Endnotes

1. *https://www.bodyandsoul.com.au/mind-body/comparison-is-the-thief-of-joy-a-psychologist-explains-how-to-stop-doing-it/news-story/e4ff079b144d743427305efa37c0d1f5.*

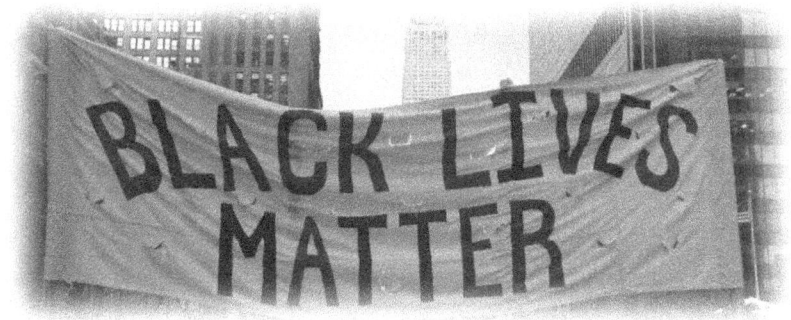

SECTION FOUR: INTRODUCTION

Societal Issues and Obligations

....

*"Justice will not be served until those
who are unaffected are as outraged as those who are."*
—Benjamin Franklin

In the fourth and final section of this book, or rather collection of essays, I delve into the world where medicine and neurosurgery merge with society and societal obligations. All disciplines, both medical and non-medical, will increasingly grapple with such as we emerge from the very tumultuous times associated with a pandemic and an escalation of social injustice. It is time to heal, but we must confront the perpetrators of evil.

Section Four

Essay 1

*The International Patient Experience:
A "World" of Difference*

What is it like to be a patient in each of the three domains of national wealth—first-, second-, and third-world environments? I can only speak from my recent experience as a patient in the US, which is a first world country. I hope to not offend anyone with this categorization, but simplicity and brevity are necessary to get my points across. I used the classification of first, second and third world countries, as opposed to High-, Middle- and Low-income countries for the aforementioned reasons. We could readily use High, Middle and Low to replace First, Second and Third World Countries. The actual classification is very complicated and, as such, I will not discuss here.

My medical problem was a symptomatic cardiac arrhythmia, for which I was admitted to the hospital for cardioversion, medication, observation, and ultimately cardiac ablation. The results were great. However, on the way I faced long lines and busy waiting rooms for multiple outpatient diagnostic procedures, unexpected delays with admissions, and significant uncertainties regarding "what next?" During my inpatient stay, there was hardly a consecutive hour of uninterrupted sleep. The aggravations were manifold. The results, however, were well worth it.

So here I am, complaining about frustrations and aggravations with modern medicine from the patient's perspective. My treatment was successful by any measurable standard, yet I complain (parenthetically, complaining regarding medical care is common in my "first world"). What I am complaining about is the result of a "first world" problem—that likely does not exist to any significant extent in "second" or "third world" environments. I now have a perspective (i.e., from that of the patient) that I did not have before.

Let me take a stab at what my experience may have been like in a "second" and "third world" environment. Please understand that I can only imagine what such an experience may be like. I have no direct experience, nor core knowledge in this arena.

Section Four

I, however, wish to highlight discrepancies that assuredly exist regarding perception and expectations in the three very different "worlds."

In a "second world" environment, depending on my financial status, I *may have* received similar treatment. However, resources would likely be limited, and I may or may not be offered all the options availed to me in the US. Lines and waits would, in all likelihood, have been longer and even more frustrating than in my "first world." Uncertainties would likely prevail regarding the quality of care, the extent of care and, ultimately, the safety and efficacy of care. Conversely, I would likely not complain. I would not complain because of very different expectations from that of a patient in a "first world" environment.

In a "third world" environment, unless I were wealthy enough to travel or pay for "high-quality" care, I would likely not be treated. Treatable "third world" problems are often restricted to trauma, and other severe, obvious, and urgent medical and surgical problems and emergencies. In all likelihood, cardiac arrhythmias (and for that matter other common maladies such as lumbar disc herniation and sciatica) are more often than not ignored and do not even reach medical attention.

I complained about my frustrations in my world, the "first world." I, however, must expand my horizons and try to appreciate the challenges faced by others. We must seek ways to help equilibrate and even quantity of medical care worldwide and to improve efficiency.

My medical problem was truly a "first world" problem. We who live in the "first world" must continuously remind ourselves of how lucky we are. We must strive to make healthcare better for all worldwide. First and foremost, this involves the provision of appropriate healthcare for all. But to the point here, physicians and non-physicians alike should all also strive to minimize system-based inefficiencies, uncertainties and frustrations. They should set appropriate expectations and convey them to our patients or potential patients. Finally, we should meet those expectations.

I fully recognize that my "interpretation" of the healthcare realities, in regions that are resource challenged, may be skewed. Henceforth, I invite dialogue regarding this subject. We all should talk it up! Perhaps through communication we can move onward as a worldwide unit.

Section Four

Essay 2
Hate: A Worldwide Conundrum

Back in October of 2018, a heinous crime of hate occurred in Pittsburgh, Pennsylvania, USA. Eleven people who were worshiping in the Tree of Life Synagogue were gunned down in an anti-Semitic act of hate. This egregious act prompted me to address the issue of hate and hate crimes, as they affect neurosurgeons and their patients. Perhaps more appropriately stated, it addresses an obligation that neurosurgeons have to their patients and to society.

My title for this piece, "Hate: A Worldwide Conundrum," is indeed applicable to all neurosurgeons and all people. Neurosurgeons are all affected by hate—the extent of which seems to take a cyclical vacillating course over years and decades. We seem to be on an up tic at this point in history, as we face and deal with genocide, war crimes, terrorism, abject racism, and other acts of hate. When the expressions of hate become more tolerable or even acceptable by a "numb" society, such upward trends are fueled. It is this "numbing" effect that we all must resist, no matter how prevalent and widespread the hate becomes. We all must resist the urge to ignore the hateful rhetoric that often permeates the news and the airways.

In these regards, we must both learn from and pay homage to Sir William Osler. His comments regarding patient-related decision making from his 1905 treatise, "The Student Life," are relevant here in that they pertain to gaining wisdom from experience.

"Begin early to make a threefold category—*clear cases, doubtful cases, mistakes*. And learn to play the game fair. No self-deception. No shrinking from the truth. Mercy and consideration for the other man. But none for yourself, upon whom you have to keep an incessant watch…. It is only by getting your cases grouped in this way that you can make any real progress in your education; only in this way can you gain wisdom from experience."

Whether physicians consider patient- related decisions and decision making, as addressed by Osler, or the curbing of senseless hate-related violence, we must learn

Section Four

from the past ("gain wisdom from experience") in order to right and steady our course moving forward. The words of the Spanish philosopher George Santayana resonate here: "Those who cannot remember the past are condemned to repeat it."

The greater than 49,000 neurosurgeons worldwide must take a stand, a stand that honors and respects human beings and their rights regardless of culture, race, religion, sexual orientation, and nationality. We all must be students of history and strive to avoid prior missteps. We must all strive to be fair, honest and to always attempt to do the right thing. We must condemn hate and movements that promote it. We must not allow ourselves to become "numb" to even the slightest of hateful actions. Finally, we must also remain calm and levelheaded, by taking all points of view into consideration.

Perhaps the most significant way we all can affect change is by talking. We must talk about our differences. We must listen to others, with whom we may disagree, to understand. We must talk about hate and not succumb to the "numbing" effects of the ever-increasing background rhetoric. We must fight back. Such is our obligation as human beings, including neurosurgeons. Neurosurgeons have an oath to uphold ("primum non nocere"—first, do no harm). All this applies to all people, not just neurosurgeons. We are all in this together.

As once emblematically stated by the Holocaust survivor and Nobel Laureate Elie Wiesel: "For the dead and the living, we must bear witness"[1]

Endnote

1. Wiesel, E. Remarks at the Dedication. Ceremonies for the United States Holocaust Memorial Museum. Washington: United States Holocaust Memorial Museum. *https://www.ushmm.org/information/about-the-museum/mission-and-history/wiesel*. 1993. Accessed 3 Aug. 2018.

Section Four

Essay 3
Black Lives Matter

"Justice will not be served until those who are unaffected are as outraged as those who are." – Benjamin Franklin

In early June 2020, Suzanne Tharin, a fellow neurosurgeon, and later others suggested that I dedicate one of my monthly Editor-in-Chief letters to "Black Lives Matter." At that time, I felt that I had nothing intelligent to say, as so many others were appropriately pontificating on the subject. I felt that anything I would add could be misinterpreted or deemed duplicative of other commentaries.

I had considered myself to be a strong opponent of social/racial injustice and injustice in general—and a strong advocate for racial, gender, and LGBTQ (lesbian, gay, bisexual, transgender, and queer) rights. Yet I felt uncomfortable regarding the expression of my feelings and opinions on the subject of "Black Lives Matter." I struggled to find an insertion point for discussion. Then, I heard an impassioned commentary from a United States American football sports commentator and analyst (Kirk Herbstreit) regarding "Black Lives Matter," social injustice and the importance of change. In his commentary, he referenced a quote from Benjamin Franklin: "Justice will not be served until those who are unaffected are as outraged as those who are."

By Franklin's terms, I am essentially unaffected, but I am not indifferent. I want to help, but how? How can I, a white Anglo-Saxon male, who has never experienced even a hint of racial prejudice, begin to understand what it is like to be an African American in my society (United States)? This is where the "rubber hits the road." This is where Kirk Herbstreit and Benjamin Franklin enter the fray from my perspective: "Justice will not be served until those who are unaffected are as outraged as those who are." Yes, I am unaffected, and yes, I am outraged. The problem here, though, is that I have not acted accordingly. I was afraid that I would misspeak (*miswrite*). The message here, from me to you, is that I am going on record as being outraged at social injustice

Section Four

and, for that matter, the fact that we even need to make the statement "Black Lives Matter." Why do we need to verbalize the fact that "Black Lives Matter"? Such should be assumed, shouldn't it? There should be no need for a "Black Lives Matter" movement, which dates to 2013, only to exponentially escalate following the death of George Floyd and other atrocious acts of racism, bigotry and hate. The fact that it is not assumed tells us all we need to know about the global perception of social injustice.

Racism, bigotry, and hate prevail, whether overtly exposed or left smoldering beneath the screen of societal barriers. What has happened in the last nearly half-decade is the erosion of the societal barrier filter to the extent that the underlying racism, bigotry, and hate have surfaced unabated. I make a case, that this is not all bad, though.

I ask the question, which is better (1) subdued and suppressed racism, bigotry, and hate, or (2) unabated racism, bigotry and hate? Sun Tzu (from *The Art of War*) stated, "Keep your friends close and your enemies closer." Knowing who the racists, bigots and haters are (keep "your enemies even closer") and keeping them in full vision allows for the development of strategies for creating change and for the recruitment of the not-as-of-yet-outraged fringe dwellers. With subdued and suppressed racism, bigotry, and hate, we do not know our foes and hence cannot develop the aforementioned strategies. Regarding the recruitment of fringe dwellers, those on the fence (concerned, but not outraged) can be identified and educated. They can be caused to become outraged regarding the way people of color are truly treated by opening their eyes to the facts and then, and only then, becoming contributors to the "Black Lives Matter" movement.

Hence, we get back to Benjamin Franklin ("Justice will not be served until those who are unaffected are as outraged as those who are.") and Kirk Herbstreit (thank you, Kirk, for enlightening so many, including myself). We need more fringe dwellers to come over to the side of justice and to actively disdain social injustice. Admittedly, and ashamedly, I may be one of these fringe dwellers. How so? Well, I had not been outraged or not at least outraged enough.

There will always be racists, bigots and haters, but knowing who they are and how they act (keep "your enemies closer") allows the movement against social injustice to pick its battles in a methodical way, while recruiting the fringe dwellers who, in a

Section Four

sense have been dormant, so that they can now emerge from their cocoon and then become vocal and "outraged" activists in the growing army of people who truly care about all of mankind.

Section Four

Essay 4
On Being Vulnerable

Vulnerability: Noun:
"the quality or state of being exposed to
the possibility of being attacked or harmed, either physically or emotionally."

"Out of your vulnerabilities will come your strength"
– Sigmund Freud

"A lack of transparency results in distrust and a deep sense of insecurity."
– Dalai Lama

"The most common lie is that which one lies to himself;
lying to others is relatively an exception."
– Friedrich Nietzsche

"If you don't understand vulnerability, you cannot manage and lead people.
If you're not showing up vulnerably as a leader,
you can't expect anyone to follow you—period."
– Brene Brown

Vulnerability, courage, strength, transparency, and leadership seemingly have little in common from a superficial perspective. A deeper dive into these human characteristics and attributes reveals a connectivity between each of them that warrants further exploration.

Let's start with the definition of vulnerability (Noun, "the quality or state of being exposed to the possibility of being attacked or harmed, either physically or emotionally"). This seems straightforward enough. "The exposure to the possibility of

Section Four

being attacked or harmed, either physically or emotionally" is suggestive, in a sense, of the notion that the exposed party (i.e., person) is weak and cannot protect himself from harm. I ask the question, can the harboring of a weakness and/or an inability to effectively protect oneself be viewed as a positive attribute? The key to answering this question lies in the difference between the harboring of a weakness and the harboring of a weakness with an accompanying effort to recognize and expose the weakness to others—i.e., transparency. Essentially, the recognition of the weakness and the willingness to expose the weakness to others is suggestive of significant self-awareness (the recognition of the weakness, i.e., being honest with self) and also courage (the exposure of the weakness to others).

Interestingly, Freud's "take" on the term vulnerability crystalizes the notion of vulnerabilities being a source of strength and courage if one is transparent regarding their weaknesses: *"Out of your vulnerabilities will come your strength."* Vulnerability, in his view, is a strength or, perhaps more appropriately considered to be a precursor to strength. Accepting and admitting vulnerabilities makes one stronger.

As the Dalai Lama suggests, *"A lack of transparency results in distrust and a deep sense of insecurity."* People who are afraid of exposing their weaknesses and vulnerabilities are not transparent and likely very insecure. These are not the characteristics we expect from a leader. Of greater concern is one's inability to "see" an obvious vulnerability or weakness within oneself due to suppression. Friedrich Nietzsche aptly puts this into perspective: *"The most common lie is that which one lies to himself; lying to others is relatively an exception."* This gets us back to self-awareness, honesty, and transparency. Bottom line, as Brene Brown states, *"If you don't understand vulnerability, you cannot manage and lead people. If you're not showing up vulnerably as a leader, you can't expect anyone to follow you—period."*

It is in this vein that I bring this conversation to the recent atrocities associated with police brutality and man's inhumanity to man. These events rapidly evolved into the "Black Lives Matter" movement—with an associated unprecedented international civil unrest. This movement has shaken us all. It has made most of us think about our feelings and emotions regarding racism. It has, in most of us, caused us to see our own vulnerabilities. "I am not a racist" is easy to say and is likely true for most humans

Section Four

who walk this planet. However, what the "Black Lives Matter" movement is accomplishing is to cause us to talk. Not being a racist is simply not enough. Not being a racist may be interpreted assuming that racism is not a problem. It is a problem, and we need to address it. We can only do this by each of us becoming vulnerable and acting on such by exposing our vulnerabilities. We can do this by talking—and most importantly, acting. When this happens, we can see our own biases. We see what it's like to walk in another person's shoes. We then want to learn more about the roots of racism and structural racism. We then can begin to become activists by speaking out against racism, educating others, talking about our vulnerabilities to others, supporting leaders who are anti-racist, and "showing up vulnerability" (Brene Brown) so that others will follow. Remember Freud's words "Out of your vulnerabilities will come your strength." Out of our strengths, will come our ability to effect change—real change this time.

Each of us, individually, should strive to recognize our own vulnerabilities and attempt to fix them, and if they cannot be fixed, we should manage them. Vulnerability management involves self-awareness and the employment of transparency. People who effectively manage their vulnerabilities are perceived as human and honest. What more could you want from the leader you strive to be. Widespread vulnerability management will, ultimately, be the key to success of the "Black Lives Matter" movement. So, be vulnerable and be strong.

Section Four

Essay 5
Right versus Privilege

"It has always been a source of bewilderment that the richest and most powerful nation in the world should have a healthcare system that, while providing state of the art services to those who can afford it and thus the most likely to not need it, either leaves the less fortunate denied or rendered destitute by the cost of care."
– Frank C. Smith, Canadian Orthopedic Surgeon

Two fundamental human needs, in my opinion, fall squarely within the "right versus privilege controversy" domain: education and healthcare. Both are, as stated, fundamental human needs, and both involve the wellbeing of individuals and of society. Apartheid South Africa exemplifies the evils that befall a nation that withholds education from a segment of its population. Generations of individuals, then, lack the skills, and health, to function at a productive level in society. They, inevitably, then become angry and occasionally hostile and lawless. They have no real chance to compete through no fault of their own.

Compound the education divide with lack of adequate medical care and the result is a "lost people"—a subset of the population with no hope for competing in society for jobs, housing, and even food.

I realize that I may be considered a bleeding-heart liberal by some. That's okay with me because I admit that I am—and I am proud of it. Such characterizations, however, are often politically derived and driven. They are, in a sense, often intended to be derogatory. It is my strong belief, however, that healthcare and education issues should not be considered political issues. They represent ethical concerns, such as man's inhumanity to man and the strengthening or weakening of the core fiber of our society. These issues are truly not "right" versus "left," but rather "right" versus "wrong" issues. We must determine what we consider to be "right" and then use politics to achieve the goal of "doing what's right." It's as simple as that.

Section Four

These problems affect all levels of society. They even affect people that you would think would be immune to such inequities. A recent internal survey* at Case Western Reserve University School of Medicine (Cleveland, Ohio, USA), performed by the Office of Financial Aid, specifically for the purpose of determining the amount of financial aid the school should make available to matriculating students, was sent to 638 second-, third-, and fourth-year medical students. They were asked two questions:

1. Do you, or have you ever, experienced food insecurity since starting medical school?
2. Are you aware of students in your class who have or are experiencing food insecurity?

Out of 290 survey responses received, 10% responded yes to question 1 and 19% respond yes to question 2.

These findings in a United States (US) medical school internal study are shocking to most. Who would have thought that such financial challenges, which seriously adversely affect education, would be found in US medical schools? Affected students often are forced to resort to seeking outside jobs to survive in school—often at the cost of sleep and study. Unfortunately, some students do not survive this onslaught of social, socio-economic, and often racially related pressures. It is likely that such is prevalent in other US institutions of higher education as well. The US is a high-income country (HIC). Nevertheless, we in the US appear to ignore such issues. The HIC environment, however, does not guarantee that all are educated, that medical care is provided for all and that no one goes hungry. Of note, in other HICs, such as Norway, Germany, Finland, France, Slovenia and Sweden—higher education is an unequivocal right, not a privilege. Higher education is free or associated with trivial costs in these countries. No student starves during their quest for a meaningful career.

Why can't we in the US make higher education, including medical education free? For that matter, why can't we treat all people the same regarding healthcare, and provide basic healthcare for all? Obama Care was a start, but more is needed. Of note countries with universal healthcare include Austria, Belarus, Bulgaria, Canada,

Section Four

Croatia, Czech Republic, Denmark, Finland, France, Germany, Greece, Iceland, Isle of Man, Italy, Luxembourg, Malta, Moldova, Norway, Poland, Portugal, Romania, Russia, Serbia, Spain, Sweden, Switzerland, Ukraine, and the United Kingdom. In these countries, healthcare is essentially free. This is not so in the United States. The clash between self-interest groups and those who see healthcare as a right is tiring and seemingly never ending. Such is the case because healthcare is politicized. When politicization happens, logic is seemingly lost in the fray, while self-interest groups continue to seek benefit.

Frank C. Smith, a Canadian Orthopedic Surgeon, once stated, *"It has always been a source of bewilderment that the richest and most powerful nation in the world should have a healthcare system that, while providing state of the art services to those who can afford it and thus the most likely to not need it, either leaves the less fortunate denied or rendered destitute by the cost of care."* Unfortunately, Dr. Smith's statement is true. How sad this is!

If we educate our people, all our people, and we ensure that everyone receives adequate medical care, our societies would be strengthened. Society members who previously did not have a reasonable chance to succeed would then have that chance.

Every year, all economies internationally are grouped into four categories: low-income countries (LICs), lower-middle-income countries (LMICs), upper-middle-income countries (UMICs), and high-income countries (or HICs). The discussion applies to HICs, but also applies to LMICs to some degree. With LMICs, education and healthcare are, overall, less available than they are in HICs. This means that the healthcare and education bars are low for most of the population. Only the wealthy can afford higher education for their children and good medical care for their family. The multiple global neurosurgery and similar projects in other areas of medicine play a role here. We must all strive to seek the "right" for education and healthcare worldwide. Together, we can prevail. Regardless, the principles remain the same, though. Healthcare and higher education should be a right, not a privilege. Period.

ACKNOWLEDGMENTS

I thank Tom Mroz for providing the encouragement to initiate this project. Without him, you would not be reading this today.

I thank my partner with the production of the journal *World Neurosurgery*, Christine Moore, Managing Editor of *World Neurosurgery*. She provided perpetual support, guidance, encouragement, and advice for the monthly Editor-in-Chief letters—which were then transformed into the essays presented in this book.

Finally, and most importantly, I acknowledge my wife, Mary. Besides being my best friend and confidant, she reviewed each essay at least two or three times, providing invaluable suggestions regarding clarity and content. One thing is for sure. I could not have done this alone.

—Ed Benzel

PRAISES FOR TODAY WAS A GOOD DAY

Dr. Edward Benzel has earned the esteem of his fellow neurosurgeons as an outstanding clinician and teacher. In this remarkable new book, he shows himself to be among that rare breed of reflective surgeons. He takes the reader along on his career as a neurosurgeon, peeling back the layers of thought and emotions that go into surgical care. Benzel not only describes what we do, but how we do it, why we do it and, in many cases, how we can do it better. From controversies in high-risk surgeries to decisions about whether to operate at all, he opens the mind and heart of the surgeon to explore the core values at the heart of the profession. A champion of humility, he also articulates the requirement for excellence. Dr. Benzel calls upon each of us to see the world in a grain of sand, the universe in our daily practice.

>Gail Rosseau, MD, FAANS, FACS
>Clinical Professor of Neurosurgery
>George Washington University
>Adjunct Professor of Global Neurosurgery
>Barrow Neurological Institute
>Chairman, Board of Directors
>The G4 Alliance
>AANS Humanitarian Award, 2021
>NEUROSURGERY, Global Section Editor
>WORLD NEUROSURGERY, Global Champions Editor
>FIENS, BOD
>ThinkFirst, BOD, International
>Interfaith America, Lifetime Director

Praises

Benzel epitomizes the role of the physician as a philosopher, as first exhibited by Galen in his book, Quod optimus medicus sit quoque philosophus - The Best Doctor is Also a Philosopher. Benzel, a renowned neurosurgeon, is not embarking on an effort to teach the technical intricacies of his profession. Rather, he is teaching each of us how to achieve "the good life."

    Jeff Brown
    NSPC Brain & Spine Surgery
    Lake Success, New York

Praises

It is indeed a delight and an honor to read the deeply-felt observations of Professor Ed Benzel, not only about what is inside the skull, but how that wondrous organ is an integral and scintilating part of the cosmos at large.

This collection of essays reveals the 'Heart of a Neurosurgeon' that is deeply imbued with awe and wonder, empathy and hope, self awareness and reflection.

Dr. Benzel may appear to some, as he acknowledges himself, 'a bleeding heart liberal', but as a man of compassion, in these essays, time and again, he is arguing, on the banquet table of history, for a place of dignity for everyone – whoever they are, and wherever they may be.

As a 'Mindful Neurosurgeon', in this book, Dr. Benzel has explored – in history, in philosophy, in laboratories, on operating tables — but above all in our own hearts and minds, the urge and need for harmony for the survival and fruition of all sentient beings, and of Mother Earth. Dr. Benzel's explorations may serve as a Clarion call for us all.

Atul Goel

Professor and Head, Department of Neurosurgery, Lilavati hospital and research centre, Bandra, Mumbai, India.

Praises

Reading this book has truly inspired me. As a neurosurgeon, I have experienced the weight of critical moments in my profession that have left a lasting impact on me. These moments include both the highs and lows, the happiness and sadness, and the anxiety and tachycardia that come with the profession.

The losses that I have experienced throughout my career have been some of the most difficult moments of my life. Losing a patient is never easy, and it is something that stays with you forever. Despite my best efforts, there have been times when I have had to deliver devastating news to families, and it is a feeling that never gets easier. These moments have taught me the value of empathy and compassion, and have shaped me into a more understanding and patient physician.

On the other hand, the happiness that comes with saving a life or seeing a patient recover from a debilitating condition is indescribable. These moments are what make the long hours and hard work worth it. They remind me of the power of medicine and the difference that we can make in people's lives.

Over time, these extreme experiences have shaped me into the person and physician that I am today: just a man and not a superman! They have taught me the importance of resilience, patience, and perseverance. They have also guided me in appreciating the small moments in life and the impact that they can have.

Neurosurgery is not just a job, it is a way of life. It requires a level of dedication and commitment that is unparalleled in any other profession requiring humanity, knowledge, and good practice.

The weight of critical moments in a neurosurgeon's life has a profound impact on personal and professional development. It is through these experiences that we learn the true value of empathy, compassion, and resilience. It is about more than just surgery, it is about the lives that we touch and the impact that we can have on the world.

Giovanni Grasso

Giovanni Grasso is Professor of Neurosurgery, Head of the Neurosurgical Unit at the University of Palermo, Italy. He is Deputy Rector for relationships with medical & scientific associations and charities at the same Institution.

Praises

In this book, Dr. Benzel advises that "we must always strive to become better at what we do." As we care for our patients and strive to improve that clinical care with an eye toward improved outcomes, we often quote the likes of Dr. Osler or Dr. Codman, anchored in our beliefs that their wisdom and sage advice will help support our statements or at the very least lend some credence to our efforts. I often look to Dr. Benzel for his wisdom on matters that separate us by his proverbial gray hairs, most of which have been long-lost on our respectively balding scalps. I have no doubt that history will validate and emphasize the underlying subtext that these essays cover, not just for us as surgeons, but as people struggling to make sense of our individual experiences in the context of our broader societies - irrespective of race, religion, and nationality -something truly encompassing of our human experience. This book will not only help shed light on the importance of what we are doing, but also give us practical guidance on doing what we do with empathy and grace. In the words of Norman Maclean, "My father was very sure about certain matters pertaining to the universe. To him all good things - trout as well as eternal salvation - come by grace and grace comes by art and art does not come easy."

Nader Hebela

Staff Physician, Spinal Neurosurgery, Neurological Institute, Cleveland Clinic Abu Dhabi, Clinical Associate Professor of Surgery, Cleveland Clinic Lerner College of Medicine of Case Western Reserve University

Praises

As chairman for 10 years of one of the best Neurosurgical programs and best hospitals in the world, Ed Benzel has beautifully succeeded in his intent – to provide insight into leadership, effective communication and fulfillment from the perspective of an international leader, for decades, in Neurosurgery.

But much more than that. Dr. Bruce Sorenson, former neurosurgical graduate from the Cleveland clinic, past president (deceased) of the Congress of Neurological Surgeons and devoted member of the church of latter-day Saints advised fellow neurosurgeons in his presidential address to always "communicate and speak from the heart."

Ed does exactly that. He has compiled a series of personal observations and beautifully crafted perspicacious essays, not only for neurosurgeons at every level, but also for laymen who are curious about the thoughts and feelings of a brilliant Neurosurgeon.

A few of the topics eloquently and succinctly explored, include: humility, selflessness, stress and burnout, empathy, mindfulness, leadership, being vulnerable, and teaching – from a consummate teacher himself.

What thoughtful person in any profession could not be interested in such topics?!

Joseph C Maroon MD

Clinical Professor and vice chairman Department Of Neurosurgery University of Pittsburgh Medical Center; Heindl Scholar in Neuroscience Neurosurgical consultant, Pittsburgh Steelers, Medical Director, World Wrestling Entertainment, Inc.

Author Square one - the secret to a balanced life

Eight times Ironman triathlon finisher

Praises

Today was a Good Day, a series of essays compiled by Dr. Ed Benzel, a consummate surgeon, teacher, and editor, is based on his experience as a neurosurgeon that stresses truth, empathy and optimism in confronting present day social issues, both within and outside healthcare. This volume belongs in the libraries of neurosurgeons, physicians of all specialties and students at any stage of their medical career, as well as all individuals willing to avail themselves of his wisdom. His thoughtful ideas emphasizing honesty, communication and listening, in contrast to those of a world inundated by the influences of social media, data overload and algorithm-based decision making, are sorely needed. Read it.

> Mark Spatola MD, Neurosurgeon
> World Neurosurgery Reviewer
> Past Chair, Ethics Committee, American Association of Neurological Surgeons

Praises

Society is indebted to persons of wisdom who put pen to paper and impart their experience and perspectives on matters of relevance. Their narrative informs contemporaneous need but also provides reference for future change, or status quo. Such persons may not view themselves as 'role models', or in modern parlance 'influencers', but indeed they are.

Dr Benzel has the necessary qualification to meet this challenge and his wide-ranging compilation covers diverse and even controversial topics to inform, challenge and educate neurosurgeons to be holistic.

James van Dellen

Emeritus Professor of Neurosurgery, University Kwa Zulu/Natal, South Africa

Praises

As a neurosurgeon with a half century of clinical, educational, research and managerial background, from time spent in three continents, each with wide-ranging levels of care and health challenges, I believe I have the experience and a perspective to be able to evaluate the substance and importance of views which impact directly and indirectly on the practice of neurosurgery. It has been described as 'The Queen of the Arts' (the title of my inaugural professorial lecture) to encompass its broad spectrum and indeed it is, but, as I have all those involved in its practice should constantly bear in mind the heavy responsibilities, sacrifices and expectations which accompany this specialty, and, furthermore, the catastrophic sequelae which can follow unwise decisions and unsuccessful interventions.

Dr. Edward Benzel's book is a profound journey beyond neurosurgery. During my fellowship at Cleveland Clinic, I experienced his holistic approach to patient care first-hand. This collection delves deep into empathy, mindful spine surgery practice, and personal growth. Through these essays, readers glimpse the balance Dr. Benzel masterfully maintains between his profession and personal life — embodying the roles of a surgeon, family man, mentor, and friend. It's a rare chance to understand a man who, beyond teaching surgical skills, emphasized healing's human aspect. This book is a tribute to his wisdom and impact on the medical community.

Sergiy Nesterenko, MD
Orthopedic Spine Surgeon
Grace Clinic of Lubbock, TX

www.ingramcontent.com/pod-product-compliance
Lightning Source LLC
LaVergne TN
LVHW012058070526
838200LV00070BA/2790